# THE
# PLAYERS'
# PLATE

# THE PLAYERS' PLATE

## AN UNORTHODOX GUIDE
## TO SPORTS NUTRITION

### EMILY COLE

NEW DEGREE PRESS

THE PLAYERS' PLATE
*An unorthodox guide to sports nutrition*

ISBN    979-8-88504-551-3  *Paperback*
        979-8-88504-877-4  *Kindle Ebook*
        979-8-88504-668-8  *Ebook*

## Dedication

*To Coach McGuire,*
*The world needs more people like you.*
*Thank you for teaching me the beauty of*
*running and the reward of hard work.*
*I wouldn't be here today without you.*

# Contents

----

# Introduction

——

November 2, 2018

Hour 1: With a pounding headache and final sip of ginger ale, I lay my head down and try to rest.

Hour 2: Everything is black, but I vaguely hear a friendly voice: "Hey Emily, can you swing your legs off the side of the bed for me? Can you tell me your sisters' names? What year is it?"

Hour 24: Half-awake, I try to roll over on my side, but my wrists are cemented in place. I can't move. I thrash around trying to rip my arms up from the sides of the bed, but my efforts are in vain. Tears run down my face. I finally give up and accept defeat.

Hour 48: Blue eyes, drowning in worry, meet mine. They are my mother's. She is sitting in a chair next to me. As the frame slowly comes into focus, I see my family surrounding me and feel the grip of my mom's hand in mine. "Emily? Emily! Guys she's awake!" my sister Julia calls out from beside her. I am in Austin for my state cross-country meet. Why are my sisters, who live in London and Nashville, here?

I'm then faced with my father's brown eyes, glossy with fatigue. Finally, I'm able to find my words. I can see the hospital gown and myriad of cords everywhere, but I ask anyway, "Where am I?" As he brushes away a tear, my dad responds in his warm raspy voice, "Hey, Em." There's a five-second pause that feels like eternity. "You had an accident."

These are the only memory fragments I have of the scariest day of my life.

**EARLIER THAT WEEKEND:**

"Are we there yet?" I joked as our van pulled up to the Mexican restaurant. Although already an older-than-my-years seventeen, I couldn't resist poking fun. Coach had hyped this place up for weeks and we were excited to be there simply to see how happy it made him. Still buckled in, I squeezed my back against the seat as my teammates tumbled over me and toward the delicious aromas of chicken and steak fajitas. After finally stepping down onto the curb of "Taqueria Chihuahua," I gazed at the colorful picnic tables decorating the lawn around the quaint wooden shack. "I already love this place," I said to Coach as he and I approached the steps.

He looked up at me with pride. "Yeah? Wait 'till you taste their food." Hunger gripped my stomach as we opened the door and my eyes landed on the freshly crafted Tex-Mex. Although I'd made this three-hour trip from Houston to Austin countless times for volleyball and basketball tournaments,

I still forgot snacks and arrived famished. I ordered and practically inhaled the hot chicken burrito.

"Sweet baby Jesus," I thought to myself as the last bite of smoked poultry refueled my tank and revived my personality. We hung out for about an hour making fun of each other and trying to ignore the growing race-weekend nerves. Unfortunately, my body found a rather uncomfortable way of keeping my mind occupied—a growing feeling of extreme nausea. Given that the biggest meet of the year was the next morning, my teammates, parents, coaches, and I were all a bit concerned, but we chalked it up to car sickness, or just not handling the once heavenly chicken wrap very well.

Once in the hotel, I chugged a couple water bottles and pulled myself together. "You're fine, stop being dramatic," I scolded myself. Grabbing my spikes and backpack from the floor, I got dizzy. "Okay, that's fine, just take it slow." No matter how sick I felt, I refused to miss the classic pre-meet tradition of jogging the 3.1-mile cross-country course with my team. Determined, I hit the elevator button and headed down to the van.

Gravel crackled under the wheels as we rolled up to the park. A giant "UIL TEXAS STATE MEET" banner glared in the sun. I thought to myself, "In twenty-four hours, I'll be looking at this same sign with a medal around my neck and a chocolate milkshake in hand." *Ouch.* My uneasy stomach churned at the thought of thick dairy.

As my teammates and I began our warmup of high knees, butt kicks, and soldier kicks, I began to quickly fade. My head ached, my eyes couldn't focus, and in the first steps of my jog, my calves cramped up so intensely that each step felt like muscle tearing off the bone. It was as if my legs below the knee were just solid cement masses. "Are you okay?" my teammate asked a few minutes later. We were just one leisurely mile into the course, but I slowed to a halt. "Do y'all mind if we stop for a second?"

I limped over to one side of the course and laid my back down on the dirt. There, I hoisted my legs up on the wall of a dilapidated shack. At that moment, I knew what I was doing looked dramatic, but I was desperate to relieve the pain. Looking back, it's unbelievable to think it never crossed my mind that something larger was going on. Nothing, not even breaking a leg, could convince me I wouldn't be able to race the next day. I had sacrificed too much. After laying there for five minutes with my legs elevated, the pressure in my calves hadn't released at all. Frustrated, I got up and continued to hobble along with my teammates.

I couldn't hold a conversation, much less jog for fifteen minutes, yet I recited to myself, "It will be okay. It's just nerves." I truly believed it would all simply turn out to be mental when I raced in the morning and finished as one of the top ten fastest girls in Texas.

## THE LAST SUPPER

The rest of that afternoon was a blur. We returned to the hotel, and I immediately retreated to my room to lay horizontal and try to keep my post run protein shake down. My efforts were unsuccessful. My gut clenched not only with pain, but also with remorse for ruining the night for the rest of the team. Everyone ordered dinner to the hotel, missing out on a fun trip to a nearby spring where a natural ice bath was meant to cap off our prerace team preparation. I struggled downstairs to grab my pasta and pleaded, "Guys! Seriously, I'm fine. Please go enjoy your night. I promise to call if I need anything." My teammates rolled their eyes at me and nearly in unison replied, "Stop being ridiculous Em. Sit down before your food gets cold." A smile crept across my face as I felt the love and support from the people who'd worked just as hard as me to get to this meet. They understood how much the next day meant to me.

"Fine. Pass me my bowl," I conceded, and opened up the black to-go box. My eyes hit the pasta and I immediately knew I wouldn't be able to keep it down. After half-stubbornly, half-fearfully trying a couple of bites, I gave in to my protesting stomach. My mom and I made eye contact, and she immediately helped me return to my hotel room's bathroom floor. My teammates' eyes followed me to the elevator, filled with worry. About another hour later, my parents gave me a big hug and left me to try and get some sleep. I was exhausted. After a full day of nausea and pounding headaches, I managed to down a glass of ginger ale, put my silenced phone on the bedside table, and finally dozed off around 8 p.m.

Thirty minutes later, my high school coach and two teammates came into the room to check on me per my parents' request. Coach McGuire could have just let me continue sleeping; I seemed to be calmly dozing, needed rest, and typically went to bed around 8 p.m. anyway. Despite this, he decided it would be better to double check if I felt okay and see if I needed anything else. He quietly approached my bedside and lightly shook my shoulder to wake me up.

My peacefully sleeping body responded to the touch by launching into convulsions, and the severity of the situation became immediately apparent. During what appeared to be a seizure, I violently shook, unintentionally bit my tongue, and thoroughly terrified my teammates. Coach ushered them out of the room and called both the ambulance and my parents. The infamous night was off to the races.

## THE RECIPE FOR DISASTER

Despite running being such a huge part of my life both in that moment and still today, the majority of my teen years actually revolved primarily around academics, volleyball, and basketball. Cross-country and track merely served as great avenues to stay in shape so I could compete my best on the court. After all, I was a junior who had never come even close to qualifying for state in either running season. Little did I know, a new discovery during the two-and-a-half-month summer break before my senior year would change everything: nutritious cooking.

I stumbled upon a few self-education sources on building a perfectly balanced meal and found myself sprinting with ease and cutting my training times down effortlessly. I felt healthy. I felt strong. I felt fast. For the first time in my life, running became *fun*. I'd been bitten by the bug and couldn't stop my newfound obsession with beating my own times. I began to utilize every part of my day to get better on the track. Whether it be waking up at 4 a.m. to eat breakfast before 6 a.m. practice or going to bed at 7 p.m. so I could wash-rinse-repeat, I behaved less and less like a typical high school senior, and more like a well-oiled machine. I executed extreme discipline in every aspect of my life for the sole purpose of achieving what had been an impossible task only three months ago: qualifying for state.

That season I not only qualified for my first ever state cross-country meet, but also became heavily favored as a top contender. I realized the energy and speed directly related to my new world of "healthy food" could help me achieve athletic dreams I hadn't deemed possible. I now had a chance to run at the collegiate level. My life was changing right before my eyes. This put even more pressure on me to continue being a "twenty-four-hour athlete," as my coach liked to say. My only regret was wishing I had realized the benefits of fueling my body well sooner. I wanted to get on a pedestal to share my discovery with every athlete in the world. This was the only downside to the huge pivot my life had taken, or so I thought.

As the most important point of the season rounded the final corner, the tables began to turn. Just as I was supposed to be peaking and giving my training its final big kick, subtle warning signs began to appear. It became harder to focus between meals. I lost all desire to hang out with my friends. I was tired and snappy all the time—and not in the typical "senioritis, too cool for school" way. This was different. It was much different.

Friends and family blamed my new anxious personality, constant exhaustion, and social absence on my rigorous training schedule. After all, I had "a lot on my plate." My bizarre eating schedule and super strict diet had me looking super fit and running better than ever before. I thought I was doing everything right. Everyone around me thought so too. Unfortunately, the emotional distancing made it impossible for anyone to fully notice the large ways in which the Emily Cole they once knew was disappearing.

## A REAL-LIFE FOOD COMA

After all these sacrifices for the sake of a breakout season, I ended up spending the entirety of my epic race weekend in a self-induced coma. During those final weeks leading up to state, I had slowly been developing hyponatremia, a condition where the concentration of sodium in my blood became dangerously low. Yep, you heard that right: sodium. In other words, I spent the most important race day of my life so far in a coma because I wasn't eating or drinking enough salt, an ingredient that is notoriously described as too high in American cuisine.

As I became more stringent about eating well, this often unintentionally translated to my food being low in sodium. That large shift in my diet, combined with sweating out salt during hot summer practices, and constantly chugging water, all compounded to cause my levels to get so low. I didn't know any better. At the time, I had no idea salt was more than just a food garnish meant to elevate the flavor of French fries. Sodium is a crucial electrolyte, an essential mineral vital to many key functions in the body. It plays a role in maintaining the balance of water in and around your cells, and proper muscle and nerve function absolutely depend upon its presence. For those who are familiar with medicine, my blood sodium level was 121 mEq/L. This imbalance caused the cells in my body to swell and cease functioning properly, leaving me irritable, tired, and unable to focus.

Finally able to piece together the blur of that weekend, I learned that:

Hour 1: My seizure-like convulsions were from my muscles aggressively cramping up.

Hour 2: The questions I heard were from a paramedic escorting me out of my hotel room.

Hour 24: The feeling of being "glued" to the bed was my parents and several nurses trying to hold, and eventually strapping me down to the hospital cot, as I thrashed around and ripped out my IVs.

Hour 48: I was face to face with my family who flew from across the world to Texas because I'd been unconscious for a dangerous number of hours and showed no signs of waking. It is still hard for me to internalize the fact that if my coach hadn't woken me up to check on me that night, it is likely that I would not be here today.

I couldn't believe I nearly lost my life simply from not eating enough of this popular ingredient many people try to avoid. This was the moment when I fully internalized that "healthy" is a much more intricate term than our society acknowledges.

## REDEFINING HEALTHY

Although my experience was very rare and hyponatremia is typically only found in extreme endurance athletes, it is a great example of how important it is that athletes are educated on what our bodies need and when. Yet, current research reveals that student athletes across all ages are greatly lacking education and awareness of sports nutrition fundamentals (Torres-McGehee et al. 2012; Webber et al. 2015). Even at collegiate levels where programs seem to have all the resources imaginable at their disposal, studies have shown that athletes scored an average of 51 out of a possible 100 on a Healthy Eating Index created by the researchers (Webber et al. 2015). By not taking advantage of this incredibly important, yet underutilized aspect of training, athletes across the world aren't reaching their full potential.

But this solution isn't as simple it sounds. Research shows an improved diet can help decrease symptoms of depression and anxiety (Matsuoka et al. 2016; Meegan, Perry, and Phillips 2017). This follows logical thinking. If you're eating healthier, you should be able to perform better, feel healthier, and be happier, right? As I hinted at from my own experience though, these factors don't always coincide. In fact, a 2021 study looked at this correlation in a much more applicable subject pool to my life: D1 female athletes. Conducted just at the height of the COVID-19 pandemic, their results were groundbreaking.

Instead of displaying the same results as studies done on regular adults, they actually found a direct correlation between a "healthier" diet and greater mental distress in athletes (Christensen et al. 2021). Although the pandemic added in a variable that is impossible to quantify, this direct contra-dictory result to the general assumption that eating "cleaner" increases one's overall health reveals the vast room this area of research has to grow. Clearly, there is an incredible amount of thought and time that must go into figuring out how to utilize this important pillar of athletic performance without sacrificing your mental health in the process.

Moreover, no perfect ratio of carbs, protein, and fat can create the same endorphins as sharing a meal with loved ones or enjoying your favorite childhood dessert. Looking back, I am amazed that the little self-taught nutrition knowledge was enough to allow me to earn a spot running at Duke today. I have since learned so much more, from reading research to speaking with professionals, and wish there had been a guide to sports nutrition for me to read as I began my athletic career to avoid all those years of deciphering it on my own; one that taught me not only how to fuel for maximum recovery and performance, but also how to navigate the societal and psychological aspects that come with fueling as an athlete.

After realizing this great need, I decided it was something the world couldn't wait for. I needed to write it myself.

Two years, countless interviews, and over forty thousand words later, *The Players' Plate* was born.

## LOOKING AHEAD

When I began writing this book my sophomore year at Duke, I wanted to make sure it wasn't just a dump of sports nutri-tion facts. I wanted to help young athletes create a balanced, individualized, and optimal nutrition plan aimed at leveling up their performance, without being overwhelmed by the science. Thus, I decided to reach out to some of the world's best athletes and teach these concepts through sharing their stories. From Olympic gold medalists to Iron Man champs, I was lucky enough to interview several people competing at the highest level possible and ask them about their experiences, good and bad, with their nutrition journeys. This, partnered with the help of registered dietitians (RDs) and scientific studies, gave me a great place to start. All the information was there; it just hadn't been put together in one place.

Every person has different needs depending on his or her specific sport and body; there simply is no one-size-fits-all solution. But there are fundamental building blocks that can be invaluable in figuring out what works best for you. The diversity and insight of each athlete made for a great layout where each person has their own chapter highlighting the importance of one core nutritional concept and how it is exemplified through their experience. At the end of each chapter, I wrap it up with a recipe that will help you immediately implement the lesson you just learned.

*The Players' Plate* is split into two sections: "Education" and "Balance," each containing four chapters. Part 1, "Education," arms you with all the sports nutrition knowledge you need to feel confident building a meal and how to take advantage of this pivotal piece of your training. Part 2 though, is what really makes this guide unique. In this latter portion of the book, I talk about "Mastering the Balance." Not just of what is physically on your plate, but in your life as well. As you may know all too well, societal and psychological challenges that come with trying to figure out what proper fuel looks like can be both overwhelming and life impeding. These are less tangible aspects of fueling that once I fully appreciated, have allowed me to achieve an improved level of athletic success. One where I am finally achieving all the dreams I set out at the beginning of my collegiate career, yes, but more importantly, I am doing so while creating lifelong memories with the people around me and enjoying peanut butter cups along the way. Essentially, part 2 gives recommendations on how to navigate these intangible pressures that may not be as clear cut, but are equally, if not more important to understand.

## TABLE OF CONTENTS

### PART 1: EDUCATION

*Chapter 1: Calling in the Pros* - In this first chapter, I interview Maddie Alm. Not only is she an All-American and Olympic-trials-qualifying athlete, she is also a registered dietitian (RD). I share all about the importance of this label (RD) in finding someone to give you nutritional advice, finding someone who works best for your specific needs, and how pivotal utilizing this resource can be in helping you find your optimal fuel.

*Chapter 2: Back to Basics* - This chapter is more of a resource you will be able to come back to anytime you need a refresher on the fundamentals. In it, you'll learn about what macronutrients are, which supplements may work best for you, and how to navigate buying high-quality foods that don't break the bank. (Think: What foods should I buy organic? What do pasture-raised eggs and grass-fed beef even mean?

Most importantly, do I need to pay the extra money for these labels?)

*Chapter 3: Run to the Kitchen* - Here, I share an experience from Lia Neal, two-time Olympic medalist swimmer to remind us that no matter what nutrition background you are starting from, learning how to cook can be pivotal in reaching your athletic dreams. I emphasize preparing your meals doesn't need to take all your time or be extravagant, and how spending time in the kitchen can be both a bonding experience with the people around you, and a fast track to leveling up your recovery and performance.

*Chapter 4: Sweet Dreams* - Marshall Kasowski, a member of the World Series Champion Los Angeles Dodgers organization, is the star of this chapter. After surviving a nearly fatal car crash, he shares how crucial improving his diet was to optimize his sleep and help him heal from this devastating setback to become the athlete he is today. With his help, I share the large impact making nutritional changes can have in maximizing your recovery at night, and which foods can help you do so.

**PART 2: MASTERING THE BALANCE**

*Chapter 5: The Mystery of Macros* - Here, I dive deeply into the pros and cons of "tracking your macros." Payton Chadwick, NCAA champion, heptathlete, and professional Asics athlete talks about how pivotal this tool was to learning how to properly build a "balanced" meal, and being able to perform better after realizing she wasn't eating enough carbohydrates to fuel her training. Despite this benefit, I also touch on how this is not a sustainable way to live, and how tracking your food intake without the oversight of a professional can lead to controlling patterns and an unhealthy relationship with food.

*Chapter 6: Aim for a B+* - In this chapter, Jesse Thomas, Stanford track alumni, Ironman champ, and co-founder of Picky Bars, shares his experience suffering from eating disorders during his collegiate career, how he has since learned to find balance in both his life and on his plate, and his ultimate athletic success because of this change. I share what a healthy relationship with food looks like, tips on how to make sure you never let your diet become something that takes away from your quality of life, and the importance of finding trustworthy people to share your struggles and triumphs with.

*Chapter 7: Social Sugar* – Allen Lim, founder of sports fueling company Skratch Labs, consultant for the Chinese and US Olympic teams, and author of three cookbooks on athletic nutrition, is the expert for chapter 7. He shares how he has observed countless elite athletes often eating alone, whether to control their food contents or simply because they are constantly on the move, and the negative consequences that follow. Through both research and personal anecdotes, this chapter demonstrates the importance of enjoying your meals alongside teammates and family, and how this practice can be more performance-enhancing than any short-term shortcuts ever could.

*Chapter 8: No More Sand Foundations* - Last but certainly not least, I bring in USA sand volleyball legend and three-time Olympic medalist April Ross to speak on a hot topic of athletic nutrition: body image. She touches on how important building a strong foundation of nutritional knowledge has been for finding this confidence for herself. In order to understand why this is important, I share studies and stories supporting how increased confidence in one's body can directly correlate to increased athletic performance (for both men *and* women), and techniques on how to strengthen this invaluable foundation for chasing your athletic dreams.

### WRAPPING UP

Although I will certainly share tips tailored to athletes who expend thousands of calories a day, this book is for everyone. Never forget, if you have a body, you are an athlete. Whether you're learning tips from an Olympic gold medalist or a Registered Dietitian, there will undoubtedly be infinite ways you can apply what they have learned to your own path and success.

I do want to mention though that if you set out to find your ideal nutrition plan with a goal physique in mind, this is not the book for you. My goal is to teach you how to listen to your hunger cues and build balanced meals to keep you sustained and powerful on the court so you can perform your best, not become a fitness model.

This book will give you an in-depth understanding of your needs as an athlete, while helping you realize that a delicious bowl of cookie dough ice cream also fits into that equation. Just as an Olympic marathoner will have a different diet than an NFL quarterback, the way *you* fuel yourself and your goals should be personally tailored to what makes you feel and perform your best. I'm not saying this is easy to find; patience will be key while you experiment and search for what works the best for you. But I promise it will be worth it.

My ultimate hope is that after reading *The Player's Plate*, you will both understand how to utilize nutrition to reach your athletic goals and feel fully confident and guilt-free when having the occasional burger and fries. As you know from my story, doing so can save a lot more than just your sanity.

## CHAPTER 1

# Calling in the Pros

———

*"A good coach can change a game. A
great coach can change a life."*

—JOHN WOODEN, BASKETBALL HALL
OF FAME PLAYER AND COACH

**SPRING OF 2019**

After I woke up from that real-life nightmare, I spent the next
few months learning the proper balance of sodium in my diet.
From carrying around a giant saltshaker my friends and I
named "Sal" (salt in Spanish), to trying out every electrolyte
drink flavor available, I did my best to make this difficult
recovery journey as enjoyable as possible. After about five
months of experimenting with which kind and amount of
sodium I needed to perform at my best, I was able to qualify
for the Texas state track meet and accomplish what I set out
to do that previous summer. I lowered my mile time from a
5:11 to a 4:50 and earned a scholarship to run at my dream
school: Duke University.

This really was a miracle considering how I was supposed to go on my official visit the same weekend I went into my coma. I literally slept through my visit to my dream college. But Coach Riley and Coach Dan at Duke believed in me and let me reschedule for a few weeks later when I had regained my strength. Their trust, combined with my track season going well, allowed me to make this vision a reality. Again, I felt confident with my nutrition. Again, I realized there was still so much more for me to learn.

Upon my arrival in Durham, North Carolina, the following fall, my training increased from thirty-five to fifty miles a week. On top of this increased mileage, twice a week we had one-hour lifts, and each day I walked several miles getting to and from practice and class. What fuel worked for me before I came to Duke just wasn't enough for this increased load. Despite all the work I had done so far, I found myself in new territory, and it was time for me to level up my sports nutrition knowledge even further. Rather than take it upon myself, I remembered that with any new subject, a coach plays a pivotal role in the learning process. Thus, I reached out to an incredibly talented athlete who also happened to be an expert in the matter: Maddie Alm.

**THE POWER OF A COACH**
Before getting into the details of our sessions, I must share why she was the perfect resource. After walking on to the cross-country and track teams at Colorado University, Maddie took the world by storm. She went on to become an NCAA All-American and multi-time US Championships and Olympic Trials qualifier. Now, she is a member of Team

Boss, an elite distance running team based out of Boulder, Colorado. When I later interviewed her for this book and asked her what the biggest change was that she made to see her rapid increase in performance, she answered without hesitation: *working with a registered dietitian.*

Just like the rest of us, she remembers going from workouts straight to the weight room on no fuel and feeling "dead." As she went through the lift alongside her teammates, her form was less than ideal and the weight she was lifting wasn't heavy enough, but it was all she could manage. Even worse, "A bike ride from the weight room to go get food was almost impossible because [she] was just so exhausted." She told me she often thought this was normal and just "how you're supposed to feel after a really hard workout," but now knows better. This can be a common misconception of what it feels like to be an "elite athlete" and to "push yourself to the edge," but when she finally was able to meet with a sports dietitian, she was informed this type of exhaustion is not necessary. Moreso, she was both surprised and dismayed to hear it was certainly not helping her reach her athletic goals.

Once she began to pack a large smoothie full of fresh fruit and protein to enjoy between sessions, she saw an immediate difference. "It was a 180," she told me in our interview, "I felt so much better. I could lift properly. Learning how to plan ahead and really prioritize fuel in that time between a workout and lift made a big difference in how I was able to get stronger as an athlete." And it showed on the track as well. At the time, she mostly competed in the 1500m, and she soon began to realize she wasn't fading at the end of the race like she used to. She had a stronger kick and was able to stick with and outperform her competitors because of her newfound strength. If this was just one particular part of her fueling that was able to make such a big difference, imagine the ways stacking up little tweaks like this can add up over time. That is what I'm hoping I can help you do as you learn the fundamentals I share throughout *The Player's Plate*.

It's no secret: the world of nutrition, and specifically sports nutrition, can be intimidating and hard to navigate on your own. Speaking with someone about your personal goals and needs can provide clarity in a place unbearably foggy when you try to go alone. Maddie's case is a great example of just how impactful knowing how and when to fuel can be on your athletic career. With her combined firsthand and professional experience in sports nutrition, it was a no-brainer for me to seek her out for advice that first year of college.

## NO SUGAR IS SWEETER

After just a couple sessions, we realized I wasn't eating nearly enough carbohydrates to fuel my body for the miles I was trying to run. This discovery has helped me to not only be able to withstand the harder training of fifty miles a week, but also increase it to sixty miles with this added fuel. It was a long process of looking at my daily physical expenditure, my current eating habits, and figuring out the best places and times to add in a pack of pretzels or an apple juice.

I am one of those people who fell into the trap that simple carbs like white bread, rice, and pasta did not fit into a healthy diet. I have since realized how each type of carbohydrate can play its own important role in fueling an intense training load. When I am running sixty miles and lifting three times a week, it is essential that I have simple carbs that contain less fiber. These provide a quick source of energy and easy digestion to fuel my long and grueling workouts. Then, complex carbs play an equally important role afterward in refilling my glycogen stores and providing fiber and micronutrients for optimum recovery.

In fact, in a landmark study, cyclists drank either a carbohydrate-rich drink or a placebo during a two-hour ride, and then completed a time trial after lasting another hour. Those who drank the carbohydrate-rich drink versus those who didn't were able to exercise and increased their power output by 9 percent more than the group who didn't (Jeukendrup et al. 2006). This discovery can be monumental for endurance athletes trying to push their body to its maximum capacity. Realizing a sports drink can be beneficial for me during a long run or workout took a while to fully appreciate, because I was initially put off by the amount of added sugar in them.

At this point, I was simultaneously fascinated and horrified by the amount of added sugar snuck into nearly every food we eat—even those I once thought were healthy. All foods that have carbohydrates naturally contain sugar, but in the case of fruits and vegetables, you are ingesting it alongside numerous vitamins, minerals, and fiber that are great for you and increase your sense of satiation (Madero et al 2011). Take bananas for example: the added fiber they provide helps slow the digestion and absorption of the sugar and curbs the rapid rise in blood glucose that is talked about in the media as being "bad."

On the other hand, most granola bars you find at the store have more added sugar than a candy bar! Combine this with the amount found in your bread, pasta sauce, salad dressings, soft drinks and even fruit juices, and it is no wonder our society is facing more and more health problems each year. Too much added sugar has been linked to chronic inflammation, metabolic syndrome, and obesity (Freeman et al 2018), and what's worse is the more sugar one eats, the more they crave it (Avena, Rada, and Hoebel 2008). These are all valid concerns and great reasons to make sure it is a nutrient you pay more attention to, but after working with and learning from Maddie and other registered dietitians, I learned this ingredient shouldn't be feared.

In fact, they helped me realize that like the study suggested, simple sugars could play a key role in providing me with quick energy for longer workouts and helping me reach my carbohydrate needs. Whether it is sugar from a banana that occurs naturally, honey, maple syrup, or from a chew, the body will break it down into the same thing: glucose, and/or fructose. The difference is the *rate* at which your body does this and when may be the best time to consume these items in relation to activity. This is why "simple" carbohydrates are preferred before workouts. Since these items are lower in fiber, the energy they provide will become available at a faster rate.

I now have bars with a little added sugar every day, and often utilize electrolyte drinks with a significant amount of added sugar for fuel during my workouts that are over an hour or in the extreme heat. Still, I understand this ingredient is something I should watch out for and try to not eat in excess. By understanding where it can be hidden, and when I should prioritize foods with added sugars, I am able to both perform at my best and enjoy the foods I eat. This is something that would not have been possible without Maddie's expertise and insight.

## FINDING A QUALIFIED COACH

Some may have never heard of a registered dietitian (RD), especially in sports. Even Maddie admitted to me that "Before my university hired a dietitian, (she) didn't know that this profession existed." RDs are the most respected and relied-on sources for nutrition information. In talking with Maddie, I learned that whereas anyone can call themselves a nutritionist—the title isn't legally protected—receiving an RD credential requires a bachelor's degree, 1,200 supervised practice hours in a variety of clinical and community nutrition settings, similar to a medical residency, and seventy-five hours of continuing education (CEU's) every five years to stay current with information, research, and literature! You then must pass a national registration exam and in twenty-nine states, hold an additional state licensure under a medical or dietetics board.

Even a brief evaluation from a dietitian can be invaluable to understanding your nutritional needs. In fact, there was a study done on this exact topic in 2017. Athletes from three different schools in the Atlantic Coast Conference (ACC) were surveyed about their primary source of nutrition information and their dietary habits. The athletes who reported working one on one with their RD reported eating less fast food and soda, taking daily multivitamins more consistently, and having breakfast before morning training and lifting sessions (Hull 2017). These are just three specific examples of how working with a nutrition professional helped these athletes. They may seem small, but once you begin accumulating changes like this over time, the results you will see in both your recovery and your performance will be exponential.

One sad truth is even if everyone knew about RD credentials, most athletes don't have one-on-one access to these professional resources (Torres-McGehee 2012). A 2020 study done at Ball State University surveyed 175 of their Division 1 student athletes asking them about where they receive their information with regards to sports nutrition since they don't have a full time RD on staff. Unsurprisingly, "the athletes reported seeking nutrition advice from their strength and conditioning specialists (48 percent), coaches (41.7 percent), athletic trainers (39.4 percent), and the internet (66.9 percent)" (Friesen et al. 2020). Although this is just one institution, it is a great example of how even athletes on extremely competitive levels are still not getting their nutritional advice from the most reliable sources.

Receiving incorrect information from un-credentialed sources can potentially put these athletes' careers and overall health at risk (Torres-McGehee 2012). Jesse Thomas, two-time Ironman champ and co-founder of the whole foods fueling company Picky Bars whom I interview in a later chapter, explained this need for more accurate health information from his own experience: "It's funny to think about how athletic programs don't let kids go in and weight lift alone because they might hurt themselves. To a certain extent, having kids make their own nutritional decisions without any information carries the same risk." Thus, make sure you remember to look for their credentials the next time you're reading information on what to eat from a social media account or influencer. If they've spent over eight years in school to earn the RD title, I guarantee they will have it well-displayed for you to see!

Though I fall into this "unqualified" category, I made sure to have this book thoroughly reviewed by Rebecca Youngs, MS, RD, LD. She is a registered and licensed dietitian with a Master of Science (MS) in Human Nutrition and has experience working with patients both clinically and in athletics. Moreover, I constantly cite professionals like Rebecca along with several research studies throughout every chapter. I am well aware that these are the real experts, and I am merely the messenger who has condensed all their thoughts into one easy to read guide. Furthermore, the knowledge *The Player's Plate* provides can only supplement, not replace speaking to an RD. Just like Maddie, having a professional look at my daily fueling habits allowed me to find a small weakness that made a huge difference in my overall performance.

One important note to keep in mind as you embark on this journey is to be open minded to new ideas. You can't go in thinking, "I can't eat carbs, that will make me gain weight!" or "I would never pay an extra two dollars for organic produce" (don't worry, there's a tip in the next chapter for knowing which foods are worth the extra price). Believe me—I'm well aware that trying to improve your current habits is intimidating, especially since the food we eat is such a personal matter. Every day I am still learning what works best for me, so don't feel like you need to be perfect either. Part of the process is trial and error, and talking to an expert can certainly help you save a lot of time. That being said, I was lucky enough to work with several different RDs over my years at Duke, and much of the basic recommendations and advice they shared were very similar. Thus, I don't want you to worry if you don't currently find yourself in a position where you can get personalized advice. Many incredible registered dietitians have social media accounts (clearly labeled with their credentials of course), that share info—graphics and tips on the most recent research in the sports nutrition world. This can provide a great beginning resource in the meantime.

Whether or not you have someone else helping you through the process, it takes bravery to seek out your own weaknesses. Of course, the fact that you're even reading this means you're already ahead of the game and ready to take on the challenge. So, thank you for pulling the trigger. Let's chase some dreams.

# TROPICAL RECOVERY SMOOTHIE:

This basic smoothie is super easy to make and contains all the essentials your body needs to either get you to your next meal or sustain you through a lift. Protein is super important if you aren't able to get to a full meal within sixty minutes, so this element is key. As for the source, if you prefer to use Greek yogurt or vegan protein, the amount of protein per scoop will differ, so make sure to read the label and get to around twenty to twenty-five grams of protein which is typically either one large or two small scoops of powder. There is a lot of debate on what type of protein is best, but what's more important is you are getting enough in the first place! Choose whatever type of protein that is easy to find and fits your needs. Lastly, the chia seeds are a great source of fiber for digestion and omega-3 fatty acids for energy and anti-inflammatory benefits, and the frozen fruit and orange juice are a great source of carbohydrates. These carbs are not only important to help your body be able to transport the protein to your muscles, but also replenish your energy stores. Drink this within thirty minutes of finishing your workout and you'll be amazed at how much better your body recovers!

**Number of servings:** 1
**Prep Time:** 5 minutes
**Cook Time:** 5 minutes

**Ingredients:**
- 1 scoop or 25g vanilla whey protein powder (or vegan)
- 2 tbsp chia seeds

- 1/3 cup each frozen banana, pineapple & mango
- 1/2 cup orange juice
- 1/2 cup water (enough to help the smoothie blend)

**Instructions:**
1. Pour your protein powder, chia seeds, and frozen fruit into a blender.
2. Add the orange juice and enough water to make the ingredients blend to your desired thickness.
3. Pour into bowl, add your favorite toppings, and devour.

* Important chef tip: for a thick smoothie-bowl consistency, the fruit **must** be frozen! This will level up your smoothies as opposed to using fresh fruit and ice. If you prefer a more liquid consistency, you can either use fresh fruit or add more liquid.

## CHAPTER 2

# Back to Basics

—

*"No matter how good you get, you can always get better and that's the exciting part."*

—TIGER WOODS, FIVE-TIME MASTERS CHAMPION
AND WORLD GOLF HALL OF FAME INDUCTEE

### KLEIN HIGH SCHOOL, 2016

It was 6:30 a.m. Aside from us, the gym was empty. My teammate and I had been going back and forth for fifteen minutes already, getting some extra reps in before practice. A single bead of sweat dripped down my forehead. Ignoring my stinging forearms and legs, I locked my vision on the volleyball hurtling toward me. My shoes squeaked on the freshly waxed floor. I braced my arms. For the seemingly millionth time, I angled my body to soften the ball's momentum, and popped it up to set and return it with a controlled but strong hit to my teammate—the classic pepper drill.

There was so much variation in this one foundational exercise: angling my arms to the side to practice an "off pass" or varying the speed at which I set, learning to adapt quickly and still get a good hit. It was a motion I could do for hours because there was always some part of my technique or timing that was off that ultimately revealed itself when I missed the ball and had to run halfway across the court to retrieve it. Over time this happened less and less, which more importantly, translated into me being more adaptable to any situation I encountered in a real game.

As athletes, we all have memories like this. We spend countless hours repeating the exact same motion in order to rely on muscle memory during high-pressure situations. Though peppering for an extra thirty minutes before practice may have seemed futile and repetitive at the time, my experience perfecting these motions helped me make the national travel squad for my club volleyball team that year despite simultaneously being mid-track season. Going back to the basics is one of the most fundamental ways to perfect your game. Luckily for us, this applies to nutrition as well.

### THE PLAN

There are several key aspects of one's diet that are highly debated. For example, how much protein do I need? Is fiber good or bad? Will caffeine enhance my endurance? There is rarely ever a clear-cut answer, but there certainly is some basic foundational knowledge that will help you when trying to figure out your personal optimal fueling plan. Sadly, a study on sports nutrition knowledge among collegiate athletes found that just 9 percent had adequate knowledge of key sports nutrition concepts like macronutrients, supplements and performance, weight management, and hydration (Torres-McGehee et al 2012). Hopefully *The Players' Plate*, and this chapter specifically, can help start to change that narrative.

"Back to Basics" covers the main building blocks all athletes should understand to be able to make educated decisions about their fuel. The information I share is gathered from some of the best sports dietitians and professionals in the world. In fact, my dear friend Rebecca Youngs, MS, RD, LD, helped review this chapter and provide knowledge that only someone with years of experience working with athletes and patients could have. From supplementing creatine to whether or not you should buy your produce organic, we touched on all the major fueling concepts. The main goal was to provide a guide that was all encompassing, yet easily digestible and not overwhelming. For quick reference in the future, I have added a Table of Contents below:

- MACRONUTRIENTS
  – Carbohydrates
  – Protein
  – Fats
- CAFFEINE
- VITAMINS, MINERALS, AND SUPPLEMENTS
- FOOD LABELS
- HYDRATION / ELECTROLYTES

Disclaimer: The information in this chapter should not replace a one-on-one consultation or assessment with a qualified medical professional. Although the information is accurate and backed with multiple resources for you to reference, a physician, dietitian, or medical provider should be consulted before starting any new supplement, vitamin, or mineral product, or making large changes in your diet.

## MACRONUTRIENTS

Commonly referred to as "macros", understanding this component of nutrition is what people largely refer to when they describe a "balanced" meal. The three main macronutrients are protein, carbohydrates, and fats, all of which are essential to maintain bodily functions, stimulate muscle growth, and prompt the proper absorption of nutrients. Determining the ratio of each macronutrient you need in a meal is something that will differ between individuals and be based on personal health and performance goals.

### CARBOHYDRATES

Carbohydrates are one of the most talked about nutrients in the health, fitness, and performance world. They are an essential nutrient for athletes that are needed to enhance muscle glycogen stores and efficiently deliver glucose to muscles during exercise. The usage and need of carbohydrates in athletics compared to its popularity and manipulation in diets seen in the mainstream media differs greatly. This can lead to false information and beliefs regarding the importance of carbohydrates in an athletic setting. In a study conducted on Division 1 athletes, only 9 percent were found to have consumed the optimal amount of carbohydrates, and 75 percent did not even consume the *minimum* requirements (Shriver, Wollenburn, and Betts 2013). With carbohydrates often serving as a main source of energy for the body, this is concerning when considering the impact on both short-term performance goals and long-term sustainability of these athletes.

For an in-season athlete, carbohydrates should be the main focus of the diet. On a game day, half of the plate should be carbohydrates. To demonstrate this, search the internet for "the athlete's plate," and you can see a graphic widely used by sports dietitians to demonstrate this breakdown. This is because as athletes, we need carbohydrates to give us energy to do work, and as the intensity increases, our usage of stored carbohydrates increases. In fact, at 75 percent of our maximum workload, glycogen, the storage form of carbohydrates, contributes about 60 percent of the energy burned (van Loon et al. 2001). If this vital nutrient is lacking in our diet, our body will pull from the muscle to break protein down into amino acids that can be converted to glucose. In other words, it causes us to tear apart the muscles we work so hard to build. Overall, the factors that contribute to the body's usage of carbohydrates during exercise include intensity, duration, the training state of the athlete, stress on the body such as heat and altitude, and metabolism.

There are two main types of carbohydrates that both serve important roles in your fueling as an athlete: simple and complex carbohydrates. Simple carbohydrates are carbohydrates with a structure that can be rapidly and easily broken down into glucose to be used in the body for energy generation. These are vital for an athlete's performance, especially when wanting to avoid gastrointestinal distress before or during an event. Examples of simple carbohydrates include white rice, white bread, white pasta, sugar, honey, dried fruit, fruit snacks, fruits, and white potatoes. Simple carbohydrates should be prioritized before and during activity.

Complex carbohydrates have a more intricate structure, making them slightly more difficult to digest than their simpler counterparts. Complex carbohydrates are high in fiber which is beneficial for gastrointestinal health and the sense of "regularity," but also important to the concept of satiation, or feeling full. Examples of complex carbohydrates include whole wheat bread/pasta, quinoa, sweet potatoes, brown rice, old-fashioned oats, and barley. These are great to have post-workout, after a gym session, game, or long run. Fiber falls under the complex carbohydrate category and plays a role in maintaining gastrointestinal regularity. It can also help control blood sugar levels and improve lipid profiles (Reynolds, Akerman, and Mann 2020). Unlike the other macronutrients, the body can't break down certain kinds of fiber. This isn't a bad thing, but athletes should avoid high-fiber foods like raw vegetables, the skins of produce, salad, bran cereal, or beans immediately before activity as it takes longer for the body to process and pass the fiber in these foods. This can leave athletes feeling bloated, nauseous, or crampy. Daily fiber needs will differ person to person.

### PROTEIN

There is no doubt athletes need protein to help rebuild muscle. This macronutrient is used for creating hormones and enzymes, involved in improving bone health, and plays a role in regulating immune function. Where the debate occurs though, is in how much protein we can absorb at one time and what the right amount is for each athlete. A general misconception is that we can only digest around 35g of protein every three to four hours, and anything above that is essentially wasted. What recent research has revealed is this is not a blanket statistic and the amount of protein your body can absorb at one time depends on your specific body type, metabolism, and overall nutritional state. More specifically, a 2018 study found .4-.55g of protein per kg bodyweight per meal to be the optimal amount to maximize anabolism, the building of muscle protein (Schoenfeld and Aragon 2018). Thus, whether you are 115 or 240 pounds makes a large difference in both your protein needs and absorption.

Additionally, a lot of people speak about the importance of consuming protein within twenty to thirty minutes after a workout, but this window of time isn't so concrete either. In fact, research has shown that a protein shake is not necessary if you are going to eat a protein-rich meal within the next hour, and that meeting your daily protein needs overall is more important (Jäger et al. 2017). This is the case no matter what sport you participate in. Whether endurance- or strength-based, a *daily minimum* of 1.6g of protein per kg helps to maintain lean muscle mass and support recovery. This number can grow during hard training stints where energy needs have increased and be higher for older athletes (Jäger et al. 2017).

Rebecca states that vegetarian or vegan athletes should pay attention to the quantity and quality of the non-animal protein sources they are consuming. Many non-animal protein sources lack all the essential amino acids or branched chain amino acids found in animal-based proteins, specifically leucine, and many athletes don't eat enough of these sources throughout the day. These athletes may need to consume more of their nonanimal protein sources to get the same amount of amino acids as their peers. Rebecca suggests including a variety of protein sources in the diet, or to look for a plant-based protein powder with the protein coming from a variety of blends such as pea, soy, hemp, brown rice, or chickpea to get the widest array of amino acids.

That being said, one lesson I learned through personal experience is it is also possible to consume too much protein. Although a rare scenario, especially for female athletes, it is possible. When I got my vitals tested my freshman year at Duke, my BUN/creatinine levels, a measurement of protein metabolism, were super high and my glucose levels were abnormally low. I was eating too much protein and not enough carbohydrates. Because of this, my body was having to spend extra energy turning the protein stores into energy, and my workouts suffered. Angie Asche, RD, speaks in an Instagram post about this phenomenon having a negative effect on one's ability to build muscle as well: "You won't gain muscle just by eating excessive amounts of protein. Gaining muscle requires strength training and consuming enough TOTAL calories," she continues. "If you consume large amounts of protein but are in a large calorie deficit with insufficient carbs and fats, your body will use protein stores for energy, and you will have a very hard time gaining muscle" or having any energy in your workouts.

The best way to make sure you are reaching your protein goals is to make sure you have a serving about the size of your fist or slightly larger with every meal. This, along with consuming high-protein snacks right after your workout and throughout the day, will help make sure you maximize both your muscle gain and injury prevention. Just as important as muscle gain though, is the ability to adequately recover after a workout. A recent meta-analysis showed that though more beneficial than consuming carbohydrates or protein alone post workout, nailing the perfect ratio of these macronutrients is not as important as eating an adequate amount. The conclusion from this study showed that a combination of both carbohydrates and protein that are appropriate calorically for the athlete, is key to enhancing glycogen synthesis versus having them alone or in an insufficient amount (Margolis et al. 2020).

## FATS

Fats are an essential nutrient that for many years were demonized in popular health culture (Vieriera, McClements, and Decker 2015). Low-fat and fat-free labels litter our grocery stores leaving the notion that this makes the food product "healthier." Rebecca states that this can be problematic, as "in many cases, low-fat or fat-free products may have added sugar or ingredients added to account for changes in taste and texture of a product." She adds that "fats are vitally important for all individuals, but especially athletes. This is because fat can be metabolized and used for energy, is needed for the absorption of vitamins, and is essential for hormone regulation and communication between cells."

There are two main types of fats: saturated and unsaturated. Saturated fats are the ones we want to limit or have in moderation, with sources of saturated fat largely being found in fast food and desserts. That being said, saturated fats are also found in animal products like butter, cheese, beef, and pork, so they aren't limited to processed foods and can certainly be consumed in moderation in a healthy diet. Unsaturated fats are commonly more "liquid" at room temperature than their saturated counterparts. They can help improve HDL (good) cholesterol. Examples of foods containing this type of fat are avocados, extra virgin olive oil, avocado oil, fatty fish, nuts, and seeds.

Omega-3 fatty acids, a type of unsaturated fat, has been shown to have anti-inflammatory properties and be beneficial in muscle repair and recovery (Calder 2006). The most well-known sources of this nutrient include flax and chia seeds, salmon, sardines, nuts, and avocado. Chia seeds in particular are my favorite. They are a great source of plant-based protein, omega-3 fatty acids, fiber, antioxidants, iron, and calcium. They have also been shown to improve heart health, improve lipid levels, and control blood sugar (Kulczyński et al. 2019). Fun fact: they make a gel-like substance when they absorb liquid, so they are great for making chia seed pudding, jelly, or adding to oatmeal.

All in all, it is important to include these "healthier" types of fats with every meal. This can be achieved by adding a tablespoon of avocado oil to your vegetables before you eat them, chef-ing up an Instagram-worthy avocado toast, or even just sprinkling a handful of nuts on your salad as a garnish. Doing so can help increase absorption of nutrients like fat soluble vitamins, improve satiation, and help with hormone regulation. For example, vitamin D, important for both bone health and immunity, is a fat-soluble vitamin.

This means it needs fat in order to be absorbed in the body (Puente Yague et al. 2020). If you make sure to include foods high in unsaturated fats while avoiding more highly processed sources of saturated fat, it will help your body feel and perform at its best while also ensuring your hormones work optimally.

## CAFFEINE

This one is for all my coffee lovers. Caffeine can be ingested in the form of a warm cup of joe, an electrolyte drink, or a supplement. It is widely utilized by athletes as an ergogenic aid. It is a central nervous system stimulant. This means it can promote focus, delay the onset of pain and fatigue, and increase the ability to perform at a higher intensity (Guest et al. 2021). It has also been found that consuming caffeine with adequate carbohydrates after exercise helps you replenish your glycogen stores more quickly (Loureiro et al 2021; Pedersen 2008).

The optimal timing and amount of caffeine is 3–6mg per kg of body weight thirty to sixty minutes before exercise. This has shown to improve endurance by 2–4 percent (Southward, Rutherfurd-Markwick, and Ali 2018). That being said, some athletes may experience negative effects. This is because people metabolize caffeine differently. Slow metabolizers may experience gastrointestinal issues or anxiety after consumption. For this reason, don't wait to experiment with caffeine until the day of competition. Lastly, recent research has also come out to debunk the misconception that this stimulant dehydrates you. While caffeine may have a small diuretic effect, it is not large enough to counterbalance the benefits of other fluid intake throughout the day (Killer, Blannin, and Jeukendrup 2014).

In large amounts, caffeine can be dangerous and even illegal. Organizations like the NCAA have restrictions on the amount of caffeine that can be consumed prior to an event. For example, the NCAA legal maximum of caffeine intake is equal to about 500mg of caffeine or six to eight cups of coffee consumed two to three hours before a competition. Once I started having caffeine before workouts and races, it took me a while to find my sweet spot. 300mg left me jittery and caused my heart rate to max out too early in the race, but I've now found a sweet spot at around 100 milligrams. I love to have this in the form of two bags of tea about forty-five minutes before I warm up for my races. Additionally, a study compared caffeine consumption in habitual and nonhabitual users at three different time points before exercising to exhaustion. At all three timepoints, one hour, three hours, and six hours prior to activity, nonhabitual caffeine users were able to sustain the exercise for longer and at a higher rate than habitual caffeine users consuming the same amount of caffeine (Bell and McLennan 2002). Thus, I avoid consuming caffeine for the entire week before my race, so the effect feels stronger right when I need it most.

## VITAMINS, MINERALS, AND SUPPLEMENTS

### IRON
This nutrient is essential for the production of hemoglobin and myoglobin. The former is a protein that helps carry oxygen to all parts of the body, and the latter is a protein that

supplies oxygen to your muscles. The four groups of individuals at most risk for iron deficiency are endurance athletes, females, vegetarians, and vegans. Women lose iron through monthly menstruation, and vegetarians or vegans often eliminate high iron sources of food in their diet. Additionally, it is very common for high-intensity or endurance athletes to be low in iron due to heavy sweating and trace blood loss in the urine and GI tract (Peadler et al. 2017). Red blood cell hemolysis, or the destruction of red blood cells, also occurs with the intense pounding that can come with activities like running, sometimes referred to as foot-strike hemolysis (Telford et al. 2003). Common signs and symptoms of low iron or iron deficiency anemia can be feeling tired, chills, brain fog, brittle nails, and decreased aerobic capacity. Athletes without anemia can still become low in iron, also known as nonanemic iron deficiency.

Iron is found in two forms: heme and nonheme iron. Heme iron is iron found in animal products such as chicken, red meat, seafood, and fish. This is the iron that is absorbed the best. Nonheme iron is found in plant-based products like nuts, seeds, fortified grains, and beans. Nonheme iron is not absorbed as well as heme iron (Hooda, Shah, and Zhang 2014). Pairing nonheme iron foods with Vitamin C or an acidic food can help increase this absorption. Contrarily, absorption of iron can be inhibited by some compounds found in coffee, tea, milk, and leafy greens. As always, consult with a health professional to determine if you are in need of further supplementation, but consuming iron-rich foods is a great way to keep these stores full.

## VITAMIN D

This is a nutrient important for many athletes, especially those who are vegan, vegetarian, or dairy- free. Vitamin D is the sidekick to calcium. It plays critical roles in protein synthesis, calcium regulation, immune response, and hormone synthesis. Vitamin D is a key part of vitamin d-dependent calcium binding proteins in the small intestine. These proteins help get calcium from the diet and transport it across the small intestine to be absorbed and used in our body. Vitamin D is needed for this protein to actually work, so this is why you commonly hear how important vitamin D is for bone health as well as calcium (Li et al. 1998). Those at risk for lower vitamin D levels are athletes who play indoor sports, have a darker skin tone, get little sun exposure, or have liver or kidney problems. A study conducted by Farrokhvar et al. 2015 followed athletes for a year and noticed that athletes were more at risk for vitamin D deficiency in the months of January and February, and in those living at higher latitudes with little sunlight (Farrokhvar et al. 2015). The nice thing is we can get this nutrient from both the sun and food. Vitamin D is found in salmon, sardines, egg yolks, fortified milk, fortified cereal, and other fortified grain products.

## CALCIUM

Calcium is needed to promote bone formation, allow for proper muscle contraction and nerve conduction, and plays a role in blood clotting. Ninety-nine percent of the calcium in our body is found in bone and teeth (Ross et al. 2001), so by keeping our bones strong with calcium consistently, athletes can help deter any detrimental bone density issues and help reinforce the strength of bones. Alongside calcium, meeting your daily caloric needs plays a key role in keeping your bones strong and maintaining proper hormone function. Rebecca states that when there is a disruption in hormonal function, specifically a decrease in estrogen, individuals are at a higher risk for lower bone mineral density (Khosla, Oursler, and Monroe 2012) since estrogen plays a role in inhibiting bone resorption, or the breaking down of bone. In some cases, calcium can be lost in sweat during activities of long duration. At its extreme, the loss of calcium in sweat could be enough to decrease calcium levels in the blood. If this happens, the body will secrete a hormone that will trigger the body to break down calcium in bone (Bary et al. 2011) leaving one at higher risk for bone injury. Calcium needs specifically will differ between age and gender but focus on increasing sources of calcium from food first before adding a supplement. This will help ensure adequate calorie intake to support hormone function and deliver a source of calcium to the body—two things key for bone health. Dairy products like milk, yogurt, and cheese are common sources of calcium. Nondairy sources include sardines, dark leafy greens, tofu, and fortified orange juices.

### COLLAGEN

This is a nutrient I learned a lot about from Meghann Featherstun, a registered dietitian I have also worked with in the past. She shared on an educational Instagram post that collagen is "a structural protein that keeps bones, tendons, ligaments, and cartilage healthy and strong." Recent studies reflect this, suggesting that collagen can help decrease joint pain and increase joint health for high-risk groups, and can be super beneficial for athletes who are recovering from injury or looking to prevent injury (Khatri et al., 2021). In an educational Instagram post, Meghann also added that it is important to consume **collagen thirty to sixty minutes before exercise** if you wish to maximize these benefits. In this post she states that "this is when the amino acids in collagen peak in our bloodstream [and] when the blood flow to our tendons, ligaments, and joints is the best." Additionally, pairing it with foods rich in vitamin C can enhance absorption even further (DePhillipo et al 2018). An easy way to put this into practice is by adding a scoop of collagen to your coffee or electrolyte drink and pair it with a small orange or vitamin C supplement before your workout. It is important to note that collagen does not contribute to your daily protein needs. We need about 2500mg of leucine to trigger muscle protein synthesis, and 20g of collagen only has about 500mg of leucine. Natural sources include bone broth, citrus fruits, fish, chicken, berries, and egg whites.

### CREATINE

Creatine monohydrate is one of the most studied supplements in the nutrition industry. It is often used in short, high-intensity periods of exercise like sprinting for less than thirty seconds and becomes increasingly ineffective as duration continues. Thus, research reflects that creatine can be helpful for sports or activities where sprints follow or are embedded in endurance exercise (soccer, lacrosse, field hockey, etc.). Additionally, it can be effective in increasing muscle strength (one rep max) and muscle endurance (more repetitions) (Gualano et al. 2012). This can be particularly beneficial for these same athletes who rely on explosiveness and quick speed in their sport.

Creatine has also been studied to aid in recovery, and decrease inflammation in the muscles. Research indicates creatine can help induce cellular hyperhydration to decrease protein breakdown in the body, It can be effective in times of immobilization during injury by increasing the amount of muscle total creatine content, aid in glycogen storage by altering the expression of transporters required to store glucose, reduce neuroinflammation in concussions or traumatic brain injury, and increase lean body mass (Rawson, Meyers, and Larson-Meyer 2018; Volek and Rawson 2004). Though there are some fears about the safety related to kidney issues or muscle damage, these have been debunked by immense research (Gualano et al. 2012). As for optimal dosage, athletes should consume 20gm/day for five days **or** 3–5gm/day for around thirty days for maximum results (Hultman et al. 1996). Look for products that contain the USP or NSF seal for safety and consume it with carbohydrates to increase creatine uptake into the cells. As always, consult with a dietitian before considering this supplement to determine if it is appropriate for you and your sport.

**BETA ALANINE**

Beta alanine is an amino acid (a building block of protein) that can be derived from consuming sources of dietary carnosine (meat), or by direct supplementation. Carnosine is made up of beta-alanine and histidine, another amino acid, and is present in skeletal muscle. Recent research concluded that supplementation with beta-alanine increased skeletal muscle carnosine concentrations by up to 60 percent (Hill et al. 2006), which provides an improved capacity to perform anaerobic exercise (Saudners et al. 2016). Studies have demonstrated that beta-alanine has the potential to play a role in prolonging the time to fatigue in short duration, mid-distance, and high-intensity activities lasting one to ten minutes like rowing or cycling (Sandford and Stellingwerff 2019). Doses of 3–6 grams of beta-alanine/day over the course of four weeks impacts the amount of carnosine stored in the muscle (Perim et al. 2019). Working with a qualified professional helps determine if this is a safe and effective supplement for each individual and his or her corresponding sport.

## PROBIOTICS

Probiotics are good live bacteria and/or yeasts that live in your body and keep it healthy and working well by helping eliminate extra bad bacteria when you have too much of it. They are great for digestion and gut health as well as immunity. A study completed in 2010 by Cox and colleagues concluded that supplementation with probiotics for twenty-eight days in twenty elite distance runners decreased the severity of upper respiratory infection (URI) symptoms (Cox et al. 2008). Natural sources of probiotics include kombucha, kefir, miso, yogurt, sauerkraut, tempeh, sourdough bread, and kimchi. Some athletes will also take an over-the-counter-probiotic supplement.

## TURMERIC

Turmeric is a spice that has great anti-inflammatory and antioxidant properties. In a meta-analysis of the effect of consuming curcumin, a compound found in turmeric, on physical activity, it was found that "Participants supplemented with curcumin displayed reduced inflammation and oxidative stress, decreased pain and muscle damage, superior recovery and muscle performance, better psychological and physiological responses (thermal and cardiovascular) during training and improved gastrointestinal function" (Suhett et al. 2020). As for proper timing, supplementing turmeric before exercise could potentially reduce acute inflammation, but after exercise is more beneficial to reduce muscle damage and accelerate recovery (Tanabe et al. 2018; Tanabe et al. 2019). When consuming turmeric either in spice or supplement form, make a conscious effort to pair it with even just a little bit of black pepper: two grams of turmeric coupled with five grams of black pepper has been shown to increase absorption by up to three times the amount of curcumin alone (Dei Cas and Ghidoni 2019).

**IMPORTANT NOTE**

Vitamins, minerals, and supplements are not regulated by the FDA. Therefore, they can be troublesome for athletes competing at a level where drug testing is prevalent. Look for the labels "USP" or "NSF" for proof of third-party testing to ensure what you are taking is actually the true supplement! Different energy drinks with lots of cryptic ingredients have been popping up as containing banned substances as well. Thus, if you aren't 100 percent certain that your supplement or food is safe to consume, always consult a registered dietitian or medical professional to make sure you aren't putting your eligibility and health at risk.

## FOOD LABELS

One of the most used words when referring to "healthy" food is the organic label, infamous for its higher price tags. Although it can certainly have its benefits, it is important to not waste money on foods that don't need to be organic. Thankfully, several organizations like the Environmental Working Group (EWG) post yearly "dirty dozen" and "clean fifteen" lists to let you know the fruits and veggies that have the most pesticide residues and those safe to eat even without the organic label. That being said, regardless if it is organic or not, a diet rich in fruits and vegetables is better than *not* eating strawberries, pears, or celery because you can't find or afford an organic version. The nutritional value of fruits and vegetables that are organic versus conventional is not vastly different, and in some cases, certain minerals/vitamins are higher in conventionally grown foods (Rahman et al. 2021).

There is also a benefit to paying for higher-quality meats. Grass-fed beef in particular is beneficial because the cows eat grass rather than grain, which leads to their meat containing more omega-3 fatty acids, B vitamins, and antioxidants than grain-fed beef (Nogoy et al. 2022; Daley et al. 2010). Again, this option may not be feasible for everyone due to availability and cost, but it is beneficial to know in case you ever have the option. Conventional meat, not grass-fed or organic, is still a great source of protein and has a place in the diet of all athletes.

One area much less clear-cut is a breakfast classic: eggs. These delicate shells are an incredible source of nutrition and contain high-quality protein with a perfect amino acid profile. Because of this, they are used as the standard for determining the biological value (a measure of protein quality), of protein rich products. That being said, it's important to note that all the incredible nutrients that eggs offer, such as vitamin B12, B2, A, B5, selenium, and choline, are contained in the yolk. Additionally, the egg white itself isn't a complete protein without the egg yolk. Though all these health benefits are well-known, it isn't always easy to begin incorporating into your diet, as deciding which kind to buy can be overwhelming. There are so many different variations, from pasture-raised, cage-free, or free-range, to white versus blue, the options seem endless. In order to understand what each of these labels mean, I've provided definitions from registered dietitian Kristin Kirkpatrick, MS, RD, LD, and a piece she was featured in titled "Should You Pay More for Cage-Free or Organic Eggs?" below:

## CAGE-FREE

The hens are not bound by cages but could very possibly be overcrowded in bars or poultry houses, giving them little room to forage for plants or insects.

## FREE-RANGE

The hens were raised outdoors or given outdoor access, and may forage for wild plants and insects, but could still live in tight quarters as the quality of the outdoor area and whether or not the hens actually use it is not addressed.

**PASTURE-RAISED**

This is the main label that actually makes a difference when looking to purchase the highest quality of eggs. The hens are fully free to forage for larvae and grubs to eat. This diet allows their eggs to contain healthier omega-3 fatty acids, as well as lutein, the antioxidant nutrient also found in sweet potatoes and carrots, which causes their yolks to be a dark yellow orange color. This is the label I personally make sure to find on the carton before purchasing.

Ultimately, she states that third party labels are more helpful, like being Animal Welfare Approved (AWA) or Certified Humane. AWA is "the gold standard" because it has strict criteria for both humane living conditions and organic feeding, but Certified Humane is a close second offering similar inspections to make sure the hens are unconfined and have access to fresh water and feed.

## HYDRATION / ELECTROLYTES

Last but certainly not least, is hydration. This foundational concept is key for performance because it makes it easier for your body to get blood flowing into your working muscles. Losing just 2 percent of our body water through sweat can decrease aerobic capacity (Sawka, Cheuvront, and, Kenefick 2005). Additionally, dehydration can lead to muscle cramping, fatigue, decreased oxygen delivery to muscles, alter power output, and impaired blood pressure (Nybo, Rasmussen, and Sawka 2014). Water is the primary source of hydration, but as my story in the intro hinted, there is more to the picture.

Drinking fluids that contain electrolytes is equally, if not more important. When one drinks too much water and is losing a lot of sweat throughout the day, their body can become depleted of essential electrolytes, like mine did. The most commonly mentioned electrolytes are sodium and chloride, but they also include potassium, magnesium, and calcium.

This is why electrolyte and sports drinks are used so readily in competition as opposed to just water. Most have a well-designed ratio of carbohydrates and electrolytes to hopefully prevent the symptoms listed above from occurring. Rebecca Youngs, MS, RD, LD, states that "the absorption of fluids and solutes, like electrolytes, occurs in the small intestine. There is a special transporter in our small intestine called the sodium glucose transporter 1 (SGLT-1) that sodium and glucose 'ride on' to get into our small intestine. When SGLT-1 transports glucose and sodium across the small intestine, a large amount of water movement occurs with it. So, to maximize how quickly and efficiently we are getting both water and electrolytes into the small intestine, we want our fluid choice to have a small amount of glucose along with our electrolytes to promote rapid absorption. Fluids with glucose are also a great way to aid in energy production during activity, especially those of long duration."

An adequate intake of electrolytes helps prevent muscle cramps and allows the body to maintain a lower heart rate during exercise. That being said, it is important to take time to figure out your personal optimal amount, because needs vary largely from person to person (Sawka, Cheuvront, and Kenefick 2015). Factors that come into play here include but are not limited to: age, intensity of activity, humidity, clothing, body mass, and genetics. On average, we can lose one thousand mg of sodium in just two pounds of sweat, but salty sweaters will need much more sodium and electrolytes than those who don't lose as much fluid. If you aren't sure which category you fall into, salty sweaters will find salt lines on the arms, legs, or clothes, can taste the salt in sweat, and may have cuts or blisters that sting when sweat is rubbed over them.

As for putting this into practice, Rebecca suggests starting your workout well-hydrated and consuming electrolyte-rich fluids throughout and after the activity as much as possible. She added that if it is an extra hot day, or you taste salt in your sweat, consider snacking on pretzels, pickles, salted nuts, or salted edamame after your workout. Some athletes (like me) may need to supplement with more concentrated sources of sodium like soy sauce, salt sticks, or ketchup packets. In these cases, an individualized plan and sweat analysis should be made to prevent over-hydrating or under-hydrating as both can have detrimental effects on the body.

Urine color provides a quick, easy, and practical way to monitor hydration status. When I went into my coma from being too low in sodium, I drank so much water that most of the time my pee was clear. I thought this was just a sign of me doing a great job, but it turns out having a little bit of color isn't a bad thing. Rebecca states that ideally, you want your urine to be a pale yellow, similar to a light lemonade, and adds that urine color can be altered by different vitamins and foods (like large amounts of B vitamins or beets) so there's no need to panic if you start taking a multivitamin and notice a change.

**WRAPPING UP**

With this knowledge of core nutritional concepts, I am confident that you will be better educated when buying your groceries or choosing what to order at a restaurant. I know there is new research coming out daily on the topics listed here, so if you have any lingering questions or concerns, I highly recommend reaching out to a professional. This can be as easy as a social media DM! You're now only two chapters into the book and I have no doubt even just implementing what you have learned here will undoubtedly have positive impacts on your training, performance, and overall health.

# PSL PRE-WORKOUT OATS

Even if you aren't a PSL (pumpkin spice latte) lover, hear me out. This snack is perfect for a pre-workout breakfast. It consists of carbs to fuel your run/lift/practice, collagen powder to help strengthen your tendons and heal/prevent injuries, and caffeine for a boost of energy and endurance. You're going to want to try this one out. So, without further ado, your perfect fall-vibes breakfast awaits!

**Number of servings:** 1
**Prep time:** 5 minutes
**Cook time:** 3 minutes

**Ingredients:**
- ½ cup oats
- 1/3 cup unsweetened milk (almond, dairy, flax, etc.)
- 1/4 tsp cinnamon
- 1/8 tsp pumpkin pie spice
- 1 tsp vanilla
- 1 1/2 tbsp maple syrup or honey
- 1 scoop collagen peptides (10–15g)
- ½ tsp salt
- 1–2 tsp instant coffee (optional)

**Directions:**
1. Combine all ingredients and microwave for 2 1/2 minutes.
2. Add water if you would like it thinner until it reaches your desired consistency

3. Add your favorite toppings: more spices, pumpkin seeds, blueberries, or even pretzels for an added crunch. Just remember not to add too much fiber so your stomach can easily digest it before your workout!

# CHAPTER 3

# Run to the Kitchen

———

*"The key is not the will to win. Everybody has that.
It is the will to prepare to win that is important."*

—BOB KNIGHT, NCAA AND OLYMPIC BASKETBALL COACH

## LATE JUNE, 2004

It was 7 a.m., but the crowd in Manhattan, New York, was wide awake. Mixed aromas of chlorine and sunscreen permeated the air. Tiny humans in wet leotards decorated the floor of the indoor facility, drawing on each other with black markers and writing "eat my bubbles" in as many different fonts as they knew to pass the time. A loud buzzing sound was followed by several large splashes and then by a wall of screaming parents and teenagers. In the middle of the commotion, an eight-year-old Brooklyn native sat wide eyed. Lia Neal was new to the swimming world and was about to head up for her second and favorite race of the day, the twenty-five-meter freestyle.

For the entirety of the early morning, she had soaked up everything around her. From observing the tricks the other girls used to fit their hair into the tight swim caps, to what time they showed up to the warm-up tent, everything was new and exciting, but one thing in particular was permeating her mind: an "energy bar." For the past few meets, she had seen her teammates eating various kinds of bars, ones with chocolate chips, peanut butter, and even M&Ms, and they looked delicious. Lia wanted nothing more than to try one for herself. Her friends were also all swimming fast, so maybe the bars would help her swim fast too. "Mom?" she asked after mustering up her best puppy dog eyes. "Yes?" her mother replied. "May I please have a bar like all the other kids have?" Her mom had also seen these snacks her daughter's peers were munching on and came up with a plan. "Just focus on your next race for now Hon," she responded.

One hour later:

Panting, Lia returned to the tent. Now two races into her three-event day, she had garnered a second- and a first-place finish in her heats so far. Exhausted, she plopped into one of the fifteen fold-up chairs littering the crinkled tarp and closed her eyes. About thirty seconds later, she heard a familiar voice whisper in her ear. "I have a surprise for you," her mother said as she knelt down. A twinkle decorated the young star's eye, knowing exactly what her mom had in mind. Lia's eyes flashed down to her mom's purse. With a smile, Mrs. Neal clicked open the snap, ruffled around for a minute, looked up at Lia with a chuckle, and finally pulled out a glossy red package.

Bursting with excitement, Lia wrapped her wet arms around her mother's neck. "Thank you!" she exclaimed with a squeal and accepted the coveted treat. It was rectangular and oddly flat, but large. The front of the package read, "Kit Kat, King Size." After fiddling with the small divots trying to find a place to rip it, she finally opened the package to reveal a beautifully crafted crispy bar covered in chocolate. In one swift motion, she snapped off one of the rods, bit the end of it, and reveled as the chocolatey goodness melted on her tongue. "Energy bars are awesome," she thought to herself.

Sixteen years later, now a professional swimmer, two-time Olympic medalist in the 4x100 freestyle relay, and founder of Swimmers for Change, an incredible grassroots athlete-led initiative raising funds and awareness for the Black Lives Matter movement. I was lucky enough to interview her for this book and share her story. When recalling this experience with me, she smiled. Lia commented about that day with her mother, "That was like our first little foray into the world of fueling. Clearly, we had the right idea, but the wrong execution." This is a challenge countless athletes and parents face daily: trying to navigate the world of optimal sports nutrition with no one pointing them in the right direction. Further complicated by misinformation and conflicting advice from social media, it can be easy to make suboptimal fueling choices with the purest of intentions. When I asked Lia what she ultimately changed to help her diet support her becoming the incredible athlete she is today, her answer was simple. It is something we have all heard before but can be difficult to know how to begin: getting in the kitchen.

## COOKING, NOT COUNTING

This was a lesson that I, like many others, learned from Shalane Flanagan and Elyse Kopecky. One of the most iconic duos the sports nutrition world has ever seen, these women are the co-authors of the New York Times best-selling cookbooks *Run Fast, Eat Slow* and *Run Fast, Cook Fast, Eat Slow*. These resources have been cultural disruptors, with their main goal being to rebuild society's connection to the kitchen. In today's world of instant gratification there is an overwhelming reliance on processed, quick-fix foods. One of the most powerful statistics they share is that of the more than 600,000 food items in the American marketplace today, 80 percent have added sugar. Additionally, the majority are also lacking fiber or vitamins, and instead are full of sugar alcohols and fillers to make them lower calorie or fat-free. With this lack of nourishing food, it's no wonder so many athletes have trouble withstanding the immense demands of a collegiate or professional career. Equipped with grocery shopping tips, details on athletic eating disorders, and meal-prepping instructions, both books provide a great resource to start changing this narrative.

Shalane and Elyse were teammates on the track and cross-country teams at the University of North Carolina, and both women talk in the books about having struggled with issues like race-weight and fueling properly. In the introduction, Shalane notes how changing her diet took the mental stress out of achieving an appropriate race weight, "Since adding more fat and whole foods into my diet, my racing weight now comes naturally—without counting calories." They share the struggles elite athletes face with regards to expectations for body image. For any young athlete, but especially those in sports where weight is thought to play a role in performance, learning how to navigate these pressures can be life changing.

Shalane gives one specific example when she was beginning her professional career running for Nike that really helped her realize the power of cooking. In her transition from college cross-country to professional marathon training, she doubled her mileage and found herself running up to 120 miles a week. As you would expect, she was burning an absurd amount of calories and couldn't seem to ever feel full. Constantly "hangry," a term for when someone is so hungry they are a menace to be around, she found herself reaching for processed snacks between meals and before bed. The fact that she was counting her calories was not helping the issue at hand as it only added more mental strain and calculation to her already physically and psychologically exhausting training regimen.

That's where Elyse stepped in and taught Shalane about the power of cooking. The famous marathoner shares in the introduction of their 2018 book *Run Fast, Cook Fast, Eat Slow*: "Insert Elyse and her nutritional wisdom, and I no longer have the uncontrollable and wild cravings for naughty snack foods... Elyse taught me that cooking should be fun and not overwhelming. She showed me how to cook with good fats to add flavor and nourishment. She also told me to stop counting calories and that the only numbers I should be consuming my mind with were the splits on my watch and miles I logged each day. Both of these recommendations were revolutionary ideas to me." Shalane has since become an Olympic silver medalist, four-time Olympian, 2017 New

York City marathon champion, third-fastest American marathoner in history, and a multiple-time American record holder. Her accolades support how athletes can see huge success just by cooking nourishing meals and eating whole foods, rather than heavily restricting or tracking their food in order to run faster.

Their books provided my first lesson in nutrition, teaching me tips like adding molasses to my recipes to fight low iron, consuming tart cherries to fight inflammation, and making sweet potato waffles to fight post long-run hanger. Like Lia, once I took this step, I was introduced to the power of intentional fueling and the impact it can have on my performance. Thus, I give a large amount of my inspiration for writing this book to Shalane and Elyse. The number of team cooking sessions I've had where we made their recipes are too many to count. I will be forever grateful for the introduction they gave me to stepping in the kitchen and indulging in all the flavor and satiety that balanced meals made with whole foods can provide.

## COOKING FOR PERFORMANCE

The feeling of being too busy to fit in proper nutrition is probably one many can relate to. It's one of the most prevalent reasons many people don't try to make their own food. I was in the exact same position. But I promise you, once you start prioritizing cooking and your health, you will never want to go back. Getting comfortable in the kitchen can be life changing, and understandably so. Studies have demonstrated an association between cooking foods like fruits and vegetables with lower levels of perceived stress and depressive symptoms (Ansari et al. 2014). Additionally, those who make the food they eat develop better cooking skills and have higher intakes of vegetables, fruits, and whole grains (Chu et al 2014; Hartmann et al 2013; Larson et al 2006; McLaughlin et al 2003; Monsivais et al., 2014).

Despite this, the United States has seen a steady decline in cooking time. From 1975 to 2006, American women have nearly halved the average amount of time spent in food preparation each day, and men have stayed stable at an average of less than twenty minutes (Zick & Stevens, 2010). To all the male athletes reading this: I give you full permission to set my book down right now and go help cook something. This decreased time in the kitchen has unsurprisingly led to more people consuming pre-packaged meals and fast foods (Monsivais, Aggarwal, & Drewnowski, 2014; Smith, Ng, and Popkin 2013). In this shift to quick food culture, we are left not only deprived of the nutrients and health benefits, but also the social connection and appreciation for our meals that cooking augments.

I also want to make it clear that in no way does eating healthy automatically mean "losing weight." I'm not writing this book to teach you how to cut off a couple pounds. That being said, if it is a goal of yours, it can be done in a healthy way, and increasing your protein can be a great way to both increase satiation (Layman 2009), and make sure you are maintaining your muscle mass while losing fat (Cuenca-Sanchez, Navas-Curillo, and Orenes-Piñero 2015; Cava, Yeat, and Mittendorfer 2017; Carbone, McClung, and Pasiakos 2019).

This awareness of the importance of cooking and eating healthy used to give athletes an edge over their competitors, but is becoming more and more standard and necessary to keep up with your competition vying for the same spots. Popular culture reflects this: Harvard Health has an article plainly titled: "Home Cooking: Good for Your Health," and famous athletes are starting to share their favorite recipes and experiment with their diets. There are even documentaries vouching that athletes need to try going vegetarian and vegan to give them an edge. Tom Brady himself has crafted the TB-12 diet, which is high-protein, plant-based, and excludes gluten, dairy, corn, soy, MSG, coffee, alcohol, GMOs, sugar, trans fats, and overly processed foods. I am not here to tell you which will work the best for you, and in many cases cutting out large food groups like this can do more harm than good.

One thing I want you to keep in mind when reading these stories or considering trying a new diet is this: although many of these athletes will rave about the increased recovery and energy from eating plant-based or cutting out processed foods, there's an extraneous common factor in the situation which is cooking more. Most professional athletes have realized they must start getting in the kitchen themselves (or hire someone if they have that luxury) in order to follow their new vegetarian, vegan, or paleo lifestyle. Thus, they begin to eat home-cooked meals with more vegetables, whole grains, and protein. Regardless of what kind of diet it is, just getting in the kitchen and using high-quality oils and produce rather than eating out is immediately going to have positive effects on your health and performance. That is why it is important to remember getting in the kitchen is a key first step to figuring out what works best for you. Your body may respond extremely well to going plant-based, whereas it might put your teammate at extreme risk for iron deficiency. Remember to always look at the bigger picture.

## RED-S AND UNDERNOURISHMENT

On that note, throughout this book, I am very conscious about reminding you that a well-balanced diet can still include a burger or hummus that has a processed vegetable oil in it. Though it may seem contradictory to the main tenets of eating "well," and the importance of cooking your own food, it is also possible to eat "too healthy." When you focus too much on cutting components out of your diet and have a restrictive mindset toward food, you can leave yourself in a caloric deficit, undernourished, and not able to perform at your best. The most prevalent syndrome of this chronic underfueling is RED-S (Relative Energy Deficiency in Sport), previously known as the female athlete triad.

The name was changed to reflect that these same issues once thought to only affect women are prevalent in male athletes as well. It also encompasses the variety of psychological and physical afflictions that come from energy deficiency. Although both men and women are affected by RED-S, a common red flag is when a female loses her menstrual cycle. This is the body's form of self-preservation: since it doesn't have enough fuel, it shuts down nonessential systems such as the organs responsible for reproduction and goes into survival mode. The main negative effect of this is a decrease in estrogen, which weakens bones and is a leading cause for the immense amount of stress fractures in those who suffer from RED-S. Whether intentional or not, this condition is a prevalent issue in the sports world, especially in those with a focus on endurance or aesthetics.

Thankfully, I have always been lucky enough to be surrounded by coaches and teammates who supported a healthy food culture and encouraged me to make sure I was eating *enough*, not less, but there are many athletes who have had a very different experience. It's impossible to tell what causes one to severely restrict their food, and the reason differs from person to person. Whether it's pressure from parents, coaches, themselves, or even external mental health stressors like school or family, no one reason is "easier" than the other. What's important to be aware of is you don't need to be underweight for this to apply to you. There are countless athletes who appear perfectly "healthy" struggling in the same way as someone who appears extremely thin. In fact, it's often those that don't appear undernourished that have a harder time getting help and recovering since it's less visibly evident something is wrong.

This isn't just an issue for elite-level athletes either. Dr. Jennifer Carlson, an expert with years of research and experience treating amenorrhea and RED-S, shared in Kopecky and Flanagan's book that the growing epidemic of disordered eating in the sports world can also be attributed to specialization in one sport so early on. She states, "There is a lot of dietary advice being given to athletes at all levels that may not reflect the increased needs of the growing and developing bodies of adolescents and young adults," and "It is a setup for undernourished athletes" (Kopecky, Flanagan, and Weiner 2016). This is an extremely important topic and yet only started being talked about publicly a handful of years ago.

In the *Run Fast, Eat Slow* cookbooks, Elyse also opens up about struggling with amenorrhea, the medical term for the absence of a menstrual cycle, for fifteen years. She shared that her passion for cooking and eating whole foods rich with healthy fats is due to her personal experience utilizing the kitchen to recover from RED-S. For years, she had been avoiding fats, thinking this was the "healthier" way to eat. She endured multiple stress fractures and thus was never able to train at full capacity. Despite some people assuming amenorrhea just "comes with intense training," she was aware that missing her cycle was abnormal. She met with several specialists who recommended artificial ways to force her cycle to return, but nothing worked. She couldn't seem to figure out why her body wasn't able to withstand the collegiate training program in the way she knew it should.

After moving to Geneva, Switzerland, though, her life changed. The food there was starkly different. Her meals were rich in healthy fats like traditionally made cheeses, grass-fed red meat, and farm-fresh eggs. What was incredible to her was when she adopted this high-fat, whole-foods diet, she was finally able to get regular cycles back and feel strong running again. She knew she had to share what she had learned with the world. Not only was she feeling more energized and happy, she was even able to have a beautiful, healthy baby girl. With women in the US experiencing infertility rates at an all-time high, 20 percent of active women and as much as 45 percent of female competitive runners suffering from athletic amenorrhea, her mission to get more people in the kitchen is one that can help change countless families' lives forever.

## GETTING COMFORTABLE IN THE KITCHEN

It is important to remember you don't have to embark on this journey alone. Cooking can seem like a daunting task if you view it as changing every meal and snack of the day. Just like Lia and her mom had to start somewhere, be proud of the efforts you, your family, and teammates have made thus far to fuel yourself well. Adding cooking with whole foods and nourishing fats to your routine will only benefit you and should not be something that causes added stress in your life. Start slow and ask your friends and family to help you pick out easy recipes you will all enjoy and can cook together. By creating a healthy culture around eating home-cooked meals and listening to our natural hunger cues, you can create lasting bonds with the people around you. In order to make this transition as easy as possible, I will leave you with three final tips to becoming comfortable in the kitchen:

### 1. PLAN AHEAD FOR EACH WEEK (SAVE TIME AND MONEY!)

A lot of people like to choose one day a week and meal prep a bunch of food. This is a great way to make your time in the kitchen more efficient and save money! By picking out what you want to eat for the week ahead of time, it allows you to buy in bulk and have quick grab-and-go meals so you can continue to fuel well without having to spend a bunch of time cooking every day. Find some recipes that make you excited and write down the items you need beforehand to make sure you only buy what you need. Another way to do this is to bulk prep a few items such as one to two protein sources, a double batch of grain like brown rice, and a large sheet of roasted vegetables. This way you have various items ready to throw together into different meals that can be changed by adding different sauces, spices, or toppings.

## 2. THROW ON A SHOW/PODCAST/MUSIC

Throw on your favorite Netflix show or podcast and you just might begin to look forward to this weekly reprieve of work. If you can find a way to make your meal prepping an enjoyable experience, it will be easier to make it a habit. The most important part is to figure out what works best with your schedule and factor in this time to cook nourishing food to fuel you through a hard week of training and life. These are the best ways to make sure you won't let your busy lifestyle take away from your fuel, or your desire to fuel well take away from your busy lifestyle.

## 3. JUST DO IT

Learning how to eat healthy in the way that works best for you is hard. It is easy to be afraid of messing up the recipe and being left with nothing for dinner, or even turning on the stove if you've never cooked before. If you find yourself in this position, remember there are plenty of resources online to teach yourself how to be safe and not burn the house down. Because of how repeatedly so many elite athletes and research studies are pointing us back to this simple act of cooking more, it is worth your time to learn. Not only will you be able to know you are fueling yourself with wholesome ingredients, being comfortable in the kitchen is also a life skill that will make you the star of dinner parties and potluck gatherings for the rest of your life.

# CHOCOLATE PROTEIN
# MOLASSES DREAM BARS

Just about every two weeks, I make a double batch of the molasses granola bars found in the back of Elyse and Shalane's book. The process of putting on some music, preheating the oven, getting out a large bowl, and pouring in the oats, tart cherries, sesame seeds, and molasses has almost become a ritual for me. It's therapeutic and reminds me of my high school days when I was first falling in love with running. Over time, I began to tweak some of the ingredients to make a product higher in both carbs and protein, and this personal rendition of their recipe is what I have included below. I melt the peanut butter and add it along with the iron-boosting blackstrap molasses and sesame seeds, and top with the salt, cinnamon, and vanilla before getting an arm workout stirring it all together. The sweet yet robust aroma that fills my apartment is almost as big of a reason for me to make them as getting to enjoy the snack itself for the next week or so. Moments like this are what inspired me to write this book and share recipes that will hopefully be as instrumental in your own health and happiness as these granola bars are for me.

**Number of servings:** 16
**Prep time:** 10 minutes
**Cook time:** 30 minutes

**Ingredients:**
- 3 cups rolled oats

- 1/3 cup blackstrap molasses
- 1/3 cup unsweetened dried tart cherries
- 1/3 cup sesame seeds
- 1/3 cup unsweetened peanut butter
- ½ tbsp vanilla
- 1 tsp salt
- 1 tbsp cinnamon
- ½ cup egg whites
- 1 ½ tbsp cacao powder

**Directions:**
1. Preheat the oven to 350 degrees and line a square casserole dish with parchment paper.
2. If your peanut butter is super thick, consider microwaving it shortly for around 30 seconds so it is more "runny" and easier to stir.
3. In a large mixing bowl, add the wet ingredients (molasses, peanut butter, egg whites, and vanilla) and stir until mixed well.
4. Add the remaining dry ingredients to the bowl and fold them into the mixture until evenly spread out.
5. Scoop the ingredients into the lined baking dish. Though I know it will be tempting, be careful to not accidentally ingest any unless you are comfortable eating raw egg!
6. Press the batter flat into the pan with either the back of your spoon, or by covering it with parchment paper and flattening it from above with your hands.
7. Once at the desired temperature, place the tray into the oven and leave for 25 minutes. When finished, the top should be slightly crispy and a darker brown.

8. For best results, let them cool first and then refrigerate/freeze them before cutting into 16 bars. This will allow for the mixture to harden and for you to have clean cut bars and less mess! Or you can devour it straight from the pan. Again, you do you!

9. Store in the freezer or fridge for a quick snack or dessert for any time of day. Make sure to not have before a practice or workout, as they are very rich in fiber.

# CHAPTER 4

# Sweet Dreams

———

*"If I don't sleep 11–12 hours a day, it's not right."*

—ROGER FEDERER, PROFESSIONAL TENNIS
PLAYER, WINNER OF 17 GRAND SLAM TITLES

## DECEMBER 21, 2015

As he tossed the last piece of Christmas wrapping paper into the garbage bin, Marshall Kasowski called out to his family, "I'm headed to the pool hall around the corner with the guys. I'll be home around 11!" Car keys jingled in his palm once he grabbed them off the counter and headed out to his 2008 Ford Focus. The D1 college pitcher relaxed into his seat, started the engine, and turned up the radio before taking off. A few minutes later, he hopped onto the 288 on-ramp as he'd done a hundred times before for a short highway stint of the drive. He carefully made his way over to the left lane, checking his mirrors and blind spot to make sure the path was clear.

Out of nowhere, the front hood of another vehicle appeared moving at a speed so high Kasowski barely had time to blink before impact.

"I thought I'd been shot in the head," Marshall recalled to me in our interview six years later. "A car going one hundred-plus miles per hour slammed into my vehicle. The impact sent my car spinning across the median and into oncoming traffic. In that moment I was a sitting duck, stopped completely perpendicular to the cars barreling toward me."

Marshall described his memory of being frozen in shock in that moment: "Time seemed to stop. I just stared at the onslaught of vehicles driving at seventy-five-plus miles per hour as a million thoughts raced through my mind... When I realized I might not make it out of this situation alive, I was almost more angry than scared, thinking, 'How could this have happened?' After years of hard work, I had just begun my career as pitcher on the University of Houston baseball team. I was finally living my dream. With that thought, I looked down at the passenger floorboard and the sixth sense came over me that I was about to get hit again."

After my own life-threatening experiences, I got chills relating to his realization that a career in baseball, and every other life goal he'd ever had, may only ever be that—a dream.

Marshall described his vision fading out, then flashing with the impact, as another car T-boned him and sent his world flying once more. A few minutes later, with several broken ribs, knocked out teeth, a gash across his forehead, and internal injuries that would continue to surface for months, the miraculously still-alive Marshall Kasowski stumbled out of his car and into a new life of intense recovery.

When I first asked him about what the rehabilitation process looked like after such a devastating setback, his response surprised me. Rather than giving most of the credit to specific rehab exercises and workouts, Marshall attributes the epiphany he had in realizing the benefit proper nutrition could have in getting higher-quality sleep. This new knowledge became a game changer in getting Marshall back on the mound, throwing with even more velocity than he was before. What could have been a career- and life-ending setback, wound up opening the door to the world of these powerful natural recovery tools.

## ATHLETES NEED MORE SLEEP

Although the importance of sleep might seem to be a well-known pillar of recovery, it is consistently one of the biggest areas upon which athletes can improve. Despite its proven beneficial nature to both recovery and performance measures (Belenky 2003; Mah 2011), young athletes seldom prioritize and achieve adequate sleep to power their bodies' physical needs. Athletes often set their bodies up for failure with late bedtimes and early alarms due to their packed schedules of training, school, and social life (Strand and Fitzgerald 2015). This already short time span allotted for sleep is cut even further by the increased popularity of social media and "nighttime scrolling" (Cain and Gradisar 2010). So much is wrong here. We cannot forget to take advantage of the incredible power rest can have in mending our bodies. Sometimes it takes a significant event, like a car wreck or two-day coma, to remind us our bodies simply must be our number one priority.

Once Marshall regained the ability to work out again, he became militant in his daily routine. He woke with the sun, hit the gym, cooked fresh meals, and went to bed early. His sole focus became helping his body recover from the trauma it had endured. Through this dedication to proper fueling, consistent routine, and maintenance of his body, not only did his alarm wake him to the feeling of his prior strength returning, he woke feeling more energized than ever before. At the time, Marshall didn't fully understand how nutrition, a consistent schedule, and dedication to sleep were working hand in hand to transform his life and career. The hours he spent in slumber became not only higher in quantity, but higher in their reparative quality as well.

In hopes I can help you fully grasp the magic that was helping Marshall recover so well, I'll share one of my favorite definitions of high-quality sleep. In a viral Twitter thread, Will Ahmed, founder and CEO of the famous "WHOOP" band, a device that tracks metrics of health including heart rate variability and sleep, broke down the most important sleep stages by contrasting two hypothetical people. Both subjects spent seven hours in bed, but the total amount of slow-wave sleep (SWS) and rapid-eye movement (REM) sleep totaled only thirty minutes for the first, and five hours for the second. "It is impossible to overstate the difference in quality of life [between the two people]," he went on. "The latter is a stronger, happier, more resilient human in every aspect of life." He continues, "Now notice I haven't yet said, 'Spend more time in bed.' The key is how can you make the time you spend in bed *more efficient, higher quality.*" This is an incredibly important distinction to realize, especially for athletes who are often busy and pressed for time.

Unfortunately, it has been found that about 40 percent of athletes experience poor sleep quality (Mah 2018). This is highly problematic as inadequate sleep leads to a lower ability to recover from training, largely due to decreased muscle glycogen stores and hormone production, two pivotal pieces in bone and muscle growth (Finestone and Milgrom 2008; Fullagar et al. 2015). Moreover, a study done on young athletes found that 65 percent of those getting less than eight hours of sleep at night had injuries and thus were nearly two times more likely to get hurt than their well-rested peers (Milewski et a.l 2014).

Although studies have shown various ways lack of sleep can inhibit performance and metabolism as discussed, time and time again, an increase in sleep has been proven to positively impact athletic performance, regardless of the sport (Watson 2017). A study on basketball players demonstrated that when extra sleep was obtained compared to usual sleep habits, free-throw percentages and sprint times improved (Mah et al. 2011).

Michael J. Breus, PhD, a clinical psychologist known as "the sleep doctor," advocates for a holistic approach to improving sleep quality via nutrition. "The closer we stick to a diet of diverse, whole, unprocessed foods, the more of these vitamins we'll pick up naturally," he states on his website. *"These are some of the simplest, most important sleep habits we can adopt"* (Brues 2022). Marshall experienced this firsthand when he began prioritizing his sleep and nutrition that summer of 2016. Although he didn't fully understand how it was helping his body become so resilient, the immense difference he felt was undeniable. He realized this discovery could be a key factor in helping him reach his childhood dream of making it to the big leagues.

## CASEIN PROTEIN

Marshall began to work with a dietitian, and more than eating a well-balanced diet, really narrowed down on the specific nutrients that could help him sleep better. As a 6'3" very athletic man, the amount of energy Marshall burned each day was incredible. He often found himself waking up hungry. This is no surprise because, depending on how long you sleep and when you stop eating, nighttime can end up being a period of six to twelve hours of fasting. For someone trying to retain his muscle and make sure he was properly fueled, that was far too much time to go without replenishing his body with some protein and carbohydrates. A simple, well-balanced evening smoothie ended up being the perfect solution.

One of the big discoveries Marshall made was that casein, a particular type of protein derived from skim milk, is slowly digested by the body. This made it the perfect fuel to ingest before periods of fasting, like sleep. "I normally had a protein smoothie before I went to bed, but after speaking with my team dietitian, I became a lot more educated on why including casein protein in this meal was so important. I learned that the slow absorbing, slow digesting protein could help keep my muscles nourished throughout the night and help me recover faster."

The science behind this phenomenon of increased recovery is that the digestion of casein protein prior to sleep allows for an increased amount of amino acids in body circulation. This leads to increases in the rate of muscle protein synthesis (Jager et al. 2017; Snijders 2019). For example, a 2012 study showed that athletes who ingested 40 grams of this type of slow digesting protein prior to sleep, compared to athletes who consumed a placebo, had a statistically significant increase in whole body protein synthesis and a 22 percent increase in fractional muscle protein synthesis (Res et al. 2012). Simply incorporating a casein protein shake before bed enabled Marshall to see both positive changes in his body composition and feel more recovered the next day. So that you too can add this smoothie to your daily routine, and enjoy a delicious treat before bed, I've incorporated Marshall's favorite recipe at the end of this chapter.

This is just one nutritional change of many that can help improve your rest and recovery. A study comparing various diet compositions showed that a diet high in protein decreased the amount of times subjects woke from sleep, while a diet higher in carbohydrates reduced the time it took participants to fall asleep compared to controls (Lindseth, Lindseth, and Thompson 2013). This leads me to an equally important before-bed nutrition topic: carbohydrate intake.

## CARBOHYDRATE INTAKE

Not only has adding in more pretzels and fruit throughout the day helped me reach my daily caloric needs as an endurance athlete, but it has also helped me fall asleep faster and deeper than ever before. I vividly remember laying wide awake in my twin-XL freshman dorm room bed, staring at the ceiling for hours on end. No matter what I tried that first year of college, from taking melatonin to avoiding screen time, I just couldn't get my body to relax at the one time I needed it to. Now, I understand my sleep struggles were also connected to that inadequate carbohydrate intake for my new training load I mentioned in the previous chapter.

There are many reasons why making sure you get enough of this vital macronutrient can benefit your slumber. Higher carbohydrate diets have also been linked to an increase in REM sleep (Vlahoyiannis 2021) and shown to increase the plasma concentration of tryptophan, an important amino acid that is an essential brain chemical for sleep (Afaghi, O'Connor, and Chow 2007). This is what Will Ahmed was talking about—getting *more* out of the *same amount of time* in bed. These facts explain why foods like tart cherry juice, turkey, and pumpkin seeds are great snacks to have before bed.

While turkey and pumpkin seeds both contain the amino acid tryptophan and thus have a similar positive impact on one's sleep like a high carbohydrate diet, tart cherry juice is my favorite staple. Not only is it a great source of carbohydrates, it also has naturally occurring melatonin in it. This is a hormone our brains produce which helps stimulate the sensation of sleepiness. During puberty, the release of melatonin is delayed which can delay bedtimes (Moore and Meltzeret al 2008). Melatonin-rich foods like tart cherry juice can be helpful in winding the body down, improving sleep quality, and getting to sleep faster (Howatson et al. 2012). I look forward to pouring my nightly glass of juice knowing it will digest quickly and help prepare my body for nighttime.

While I know some of you might want to use this as an excuse to indulge in your favorite dessert after dinner, I hate to break it to you that not all carbohydrates are created equally. A 2022 study found a positive correlation between high levels of added sugar intake and poor quality of sleep (Alahmary et al. 2022). Timing is everything when consuming simple sugars, and the hours right before bed are when they should be avoided (Alamary et al. 2022).

## SWEET DREAMS

Despite the many food options you now know that can help you get better sleep, I am well aware that sometimes no snack is strong enough to mitigate the impacts of adrenalin and a racing heart rate from a late-night high-stress game or practice.

Marshall experienced this in one of the most extreme forms imaginable: minor league baseball. For those who don't know, baseball athletes typically spend years playing in one of the four minor league divisions: low A, high A, double A, and triple A before eventually quitting (90 percent) or getting called up to the major leagues (10 percent). This process is grueling: after graduating, Marshall spent the next three years grinding his way through the minor leagues with wages near poverty level (Gordon 2014). On top of his one-hundred-hour-plus training week, he found himself working other side jobs well into the night in order to pay bills.

This sacrifice didn't deter Marshall. Confident in his abilities, he was never phased from chasing this dream. In a new position as a relieving pitcher, he enjoyed the learning that came with every day, but faced a large new dilemma: the excitement of coming in late to close out the win made trying to sleep a nightmare. In this role, Marshall entered the game typically anywhere from 9–12 p.m. Right about when most people are crawling in bed with a good book, Marshall expected to be primed for peak performance. And no matter how many remedies he tried, the young star would inevitably return home wired and unable to fall asleep.

One particular game in Tulsa, Oklahoma, that he was put in to close stood out when I asked him about this struggle. With some movement in the big leagues and having played well for the past month, Marshall knew all eyes were on him. He took a deep breath, looked around at the stands, and knew this was his moment. One by one, he struck out the next three batters. Adrenaline and excitement coursed through his body as he realized the game was over and he'd done exactly what he needed. Finally, after all the hard work to come back from the car crash, getting that call up to the big leagues seemed like a reality. He recalled, "I tried to go to bed that night and I just remember thinking 'There's absolutely no way I'm falling asleep.' I just stared at my phone, waiting for it to ring, and probably didn't go to bed until 4:30 that morning." Afterward, he began to work with his team dietitian again on more tactics to wind down before bed and potential supplements that could help him avoid another sleepless night. This is where he learned about the power of taking a magnesium supplement before bed.

Performing a different role than melatonin, low levels of this important micronutrient are associated with poor sleep quality and insomnia (Djokic et al. 2019). This could be a key discovery as it appears most athletes do not consume enough magnesium in their diets (Volpe 2015). As always, getting your daily requirement of this nutrient through whole foods is more ideal than taking a supplement, but some athletes may see benefits from consuming it in various forms. There are plenty of foods rich in this nutrient: leafy green vegetables, nuts and seeds, whole grains, yogurt and milk, and even soy products. He began to incorporate these as well as a magnesium supplement before bed into his diet, along with a good wind-down routine once arriving home. Again, Marshall was able to see his sleep improve along with his game. With more consistent performances and an even better understanding of what he needed as an athlete, he finally received the long-awaited phone call. The Texas native was invited to join the big-league spring training camp with the Los Angeles Dodgers in January 2020.

**SLEEP TIPS SUMMARY:**

Whether Marshall is winding up in front of a crowd of thousands or winding down in the comfort of his bedroom, he now knows how to fuel himself properly to get the most out of his sleep. He vouches that this has been a secret ingredient to his athletic success, and I have felt similar incredible changes in my performance from optimizing this pillar of my training. Just as he had specific discoveries that allowed him to sleep better, you will experience unique changes that are beneficial to you. Hopefully reading through our experiences can help point you in the direction of success. I'm pumped for you to try out these new tips and feel the immediate benefit that high quality sleep can have on your performance and life in general. If there's one thing Marshall's journey should teach you, it's to never count yourself out of your biggest dreams. Who knows—if you really take these sleep tips to heart, you just might wake up one day and find yourself a World Series Champion.

Best practices:

- Cold room (65 degrees)
- No blue light two hours before bed (or use blue light glasses if you must)
- Limit processed sugars and heavy meals late at night
- Consider taking magnesium or melatonin supplement
- Take a warm shower
- Read a book and wind down for thirty to sixty minutes before desired bedtime

Snack ideas: tart cherry juice, turkey, pumpkin seeds, casein protein shake

# MARSHALL'S FAVORITE BEDTIME SMOOTHIE

Perfect for refueling carbs and protein stores before you go to bed, Marshall's super easy sleep-enhancing smoothie is one you don't want to miss out on. The slow-release casein will provide protein over a longer period of time, thus making it a top-tier recipe for overnight recovery!

**Number of servings:** 1
**Prep time:** 5 minutes
**Cook time:** 2 minutes

**Ingredients:**
- 1 large banana (freeze ahead of time for a more thick consistency)
- 1 scoop (29g) chocolate protein powder*
- 1 scoop (29g) casein protein powder
- 1 cup grass fed milk
- 1 cup water
- 1 tbsp almond butter
- 1 cup of ice

**Directions:**
1. Throw all ingredients in a blender, and blend until you reach your desired consistency
2. Pour into a cup and add your favorite toppings (ideas: granola, chocolate chips, pumpkin seeds)

*If you have lower protein needs, just leave out the extra scoop of regular protein powder!

## CHAPTER 5

# The Mystery of Macros

—

*"I stopped trying to do a great many difficult things perfectly because it had become clear in my mind that this ambitious over-thoroughness was neither possible nor advisable, or even necessary."*

—BEN HOGAN, HALL OF FAME AMERICAN GOLFER

## JUNE 6, 2019

Another bead of sweat crawled down my face. Amused at this point, I stuck out my tongue and laughed as the salty drop landed in my mouth. Home sweet home. The crowd around me roared as the long jump competition went on in front of my section in the stands at the University of Texas. I had just been here to compete in the Texas state high school track meet, but this time I was a spectator watching the next level in a meet I dreamed of getting to be a part of: the 2019 NCAA outdoor track and field championships. I cupped my hand over my eyes to block the sun and peered over the rainbow of college uniforms decorating the athletes in front of me.

"There she is!" I whispered as I nudged my dad and pointed. On the track, a pristine white singlet flashed under a wave of blond hair.

Payton Chadwick, 2018 NCAA national champion in the 60-meter hurdles jumped around on the track in front of us to keep warm. With each step, her legs rippled to display every individual muscle in her quads. She was undeniably impressive. Where most people were happy to be competing in this championship meet in one event, she ended up not only qualifying for, but earning first team All-American honors in both the 4x100-meter relay and 100-meter hurdles. What's more is that in prior years she had specialized in an arguably more difficult feat: the heptathlon.

For those who don't know, the women's heptathlon is one of the most impressive displays of athleticism in any sport: this event is a compilation of *seven* different track events over *two* days. On day one, athletes compete in the 100-meter hurdles, high jump, shot put, and 200-meter run. Then, they proceed to double back the next day for the long jump, javelin throw, and 800-meter run. Clearly, these athletes must be incredibly physically and mentally strong. Even among this high caliber crowd though, Payton rose to the top. During her collegiate career, she garnered twelve first team All-American accolades, set school records in the 60-meter hurdles and the 4x100-meter relay, and as I mentioned above, was a national champion in 2018. If those accomplishments are a mouthful to read, imagine going through the effort to actually achieve all of them.

Thus, when I watched her from the metal stands that hot summer afternoon, I was immediately intrigued about how her diet has played a role in such a successful career. A year and a half later when I began to write this book, I knew I wanted her to be a part of it. Now a professional athlete for Asics, she had a couple more years of training and experience under her belt and was happy to share with me what all she had learned. When I asked her what one thing she wished she had known earlier in her career, she had a surprising answer: the power of tracking your macros.

## THE RESEARCH

"Tracking your macros" is a phrase you may have heard before from fitness brands or influencers. For those familiar with the subject, bear with me while I catch the rest of us up to speed. Macronutrients are defined by the World Health Organization as "nutrients that provide calories or energy and are required in large amounts to maintain body functions and carry out the activities of daily life," while micronutrients are those that we require in smaller amounts, like vitamins and minerals. There are three main macronutrients: carbohydrates, proteins, and fats. Therefore, all that "tracking your macros" means is measuring and making sure you are getting the proper ratio of these nutrients each day, and at each meal. There have been very mixed reviews on this method of eating, some raving about the performance and physique gains it provides and others being adamant and apprehensive of the disordered eating patterns it encourages.

On one hand, for an athlete needing to gain weight or make weight for their sport, carb load before a marathon may benefit and feel comforted by tracking macros, but this practice isn't always beneficial. In fact, studies reveal athletes who are asked to track food may inaccurately report the types of foods they eat in order to impress others. There is likely to be biased reporting toward healthier foods like produce, and away from sugar or fat-filled foods (Worsley et al. 1984, Macdiarmid and Blundeel 1997). Furthermore, many people will not get accurate macronutrient breakdowns from an online calculator or app. For example, an athlete trying to run a PR in a cross-country meet should have a pre-race meal or snack primarily comprised of simple carbohydrates, but this could go over their allotted macronutrients for the day based on what their app says.

Another example of when counting macros may not be helpful is when an athlete is trying to recover from an injury or regain a menstrual cycle. Rebecca Youngs, MS, RD, LD, states, "Calorie intake, healthy fats, and the caloric density of foods are extremely important factors when working with an athlete who is trying to re-establish a menstrual cycle. More specifically, a pre-set number of calories and macronutrients will not take into account the possible effect of fat intake on hormone regulation." Having a general understanding of what each macronutrient is, when to have it, and how it makes you feel is important, but letting numbers dictate what and when to eat can be a slippery slope. Rebecca suggests focusing on other aspects of health and performance to determine if you are getting the best ratio of macros such as energy levels at practice, the ability to recover from a workout, or having a monthly menstrual cycle.

## WEIGHING THE PROS AND CONS

Maddie Alm, the professional runner and registered dietitian from chapter 1, had a similar viewpoint on the benefits and detriments of tracking in my interview with her: "It depends on why you're doing it, and where you're getting your numbers from. If you're doing it to just check in once in a while and make sure you're eating enough, that's one thing. If you're doing it religiously, it's starting to cause you to feel obsessed with your food, or you feel guilty if you go over on certain things, that is when it becomes an issue. Also, the problem with a lot of those programs that give you macros is their estimations are very off, so if you're going to track macros you're much better off doing it with a registered dietitian who can calculate your exact needs and help you navigate it in a way that doesn't harm your relationship with food. It is not something I usually recommend doing, especially not on your own." There are two completely different experiences one can have with this way of eating, experiences that both Payton and I have had.

The first example is where you follow this plan for a short amount of time and love it. You learn a lot about your current eating habits and how to build a balanced meal, perhaps even see some physique or performance gains because of it. You're able to make sure you're still hitting your overall caloric needs because you are in a controlled environment, like having your own kitchen and fridge and being able to cook all your own meals with no added stress.

The latter is where you try to maintain this way of eating beyond this initial learning phase into a busy lifestyle where you may have to eat out or travel for competitions, and it begins to take over your life. All of a sudden, 80 percent of your brain power is consumed calculating what you will eat for your next meal, which inevitably negatively affects your performance, relationships, and mental health.

## THE FIRST SCENARIO

Despite the potential downsides, Payton is someone who has felt prior, positive experience with this nutrition technique. She shared that growing up, both her parents were very sports- and nutrition-oriented, but that didn't mean she fully understood how to properly fuel. The NCAA champ admitted, "In my house, we did not have bad foods." Every morning, she would wake up to the smell of buttered toast and scrambled eggs along with fresh juices made by her dad to wash it down. It was a dream setup for fueling her intense training; she got all the benefits of home-cooked meals without having to spend the time make them herself. Despite this great variety of healthy nutrients, this later came at a cost. She looks back now and states that though she was giving her body what it needed, she didn't fully learn how to build a properly balanced plate of carbs, protein, and fat *by herself.* This lack of knowledge on how to properly fuel on her own was made evident when she got to college and didn't have anyone guiding her nutritionally anymore.

She ended up trying both the keto and paleo diets, and now greatly discourages any other athletes from trying these paths as she did. "I had always thought carbs were the devil, so I would try and stay away from them," she said. "I would grab an Unwich from Jimmy Johns (a sandwich with a lettuce wrap instead of a bun), and thirty minutes later, I was starving." This experience was from testing the ketogenic diet, which is known for its zero-tolerance policy on carbs and was originally created to treat children with epileptic seizures in the early 1900s. Payton shares that even when she transitioned to the paleo diet during the outdoor track season of 2017, it contained nearly no carbs as well. This latter diet is meant to mimic the hunter-gatherer lifestyle before farming, and consists mainly of whole foods, fruits and vegetables, fresh proteins, and healthy fats.

Though this is a great base for a healthy diet, it limits dairy, grains, and legumes, which has caused a lot of controversy, and makes it especially difficult for athletes to meet their carbohydrate needs. Payton shared a memory with me where she had "zero energy" when trying to complete a workout that was typically her favorite. After seeing how difficult every action of the practice was, her coach even bluntly asked, "What is wrong with you?" She had no idea at the time that this lethargy was largely due to her being in carb depletion. "I just was not getting the proper nutrition," she reflected. "Now after I eat something with the right amount of carbs, I feel full for hours after and am more energized for practice than ever before."

What Payton enjoys most about this way of fueling is for her, it is not another fad diet. It is an understanding of how much of each nutrient her body needs at each point in the day to maximize her recovery and enhance her energy levels. Not only has she been able to see huge performance and physical changes simply from giving her body the proper ratio of macronutrients, but she also realized she can and should eat much more food to properly recover. She recalled when she first began tracking: "I was like, 'Oh my gosh, I can't eat that much. That's so much food!' But then I started doing it. And while I was training during the quarantine time of the 2019 Coronavirus epidemic, I had so much more energy and I was able to maintain my weight. This has just never felt like a diet; that's why I like it."

## THE SECOND SCENARIO

My own journey was a similar experience at first. Most of my initial knowledge around proper nutrition came from tracking my macros, but it ultimately became burdensome to both my mental health and performance. I was a junior in high school, and just getting into track season after finishing off my last basketball playoff game. I distinctly remember one day scrolling through the "health" section off the app store. At the time, I had no desire to lose weight or any idea of what a macronutrient was, but one particular app looked cool, so I thought, 'Why not try it out?' It ended up being one that helped you track your macros, and I set to the muscle building setting. Each meal was anywhere from 50–75g carbs, 20–30g fat, 40g protein, at least 8g fiber, and less than 7g added sugar. I was fascinated. It was fun for me to see how, just like Payton, I could eat *such* a large volume of healthy food, and never feel bogged down as if I had eaten too much.

Up until that point, I had eaten poorly with no sense of "mealtimes" or "balance." I had countless late-night study sessions after sports games where I was grinding away at my desk and suddenly hit with a pang of hunger. I would routinely go downstairs around 1 a.m., turn on the kitchen light, and pour a bowl of fruity rice cereal. Of course, this was never satiating, so I often had two to four bowls at a time, and then went back upstairs to keep working until either I finished or I fell asleep at my desk. Once I began to track my macros and fully comprehend just how much better I could wake up feeling the next day had I chosen a healthier, more balanced snack, my whole life began to change. Where the sugar-dense cereal used to leave me bloated and unsatisfied, homemade granola bars and date balls provided me with sustained energy and a happy digestive system.

I was running like I never had before in practice and starting to lean out—all while still having no real intention of doing so. I was just tracking because I liked to know what was going into each meal, and all of a sudden, two months later, I looked in the mirror and didn't recognize the girl staring back at me. Where I before had seen a normal eighteen-year-old body, I now saw someone with ripped arms and even a hint of abs. I had both lost weight and drastically changed my body composition and to be honest, didn't really understand how. All I knew was that I was balancing my carbs, protein, and fat at each meal, and eating around 150 g of protein each day. I had my debut for cross-country season at the Marcus 1 meet in Dallas, Texas. Here, I ran an 18:13 5k, smashing my PR from the previous year by nearly two minutes—and couldn't wait to continue on the season with my "secret recipe" to success. That was when the shine started to slowly wear off.

As school started and classes picked up, I had less and less time to worry about the food that was going into my body. I wasn't good about meal prepping and I was trying to balance six-in-the-morning track workouts with six AP classes and staying on my schedule of four to five smaller, high-protein meals throughout the day. I wore myself thin, no pun intended, trying to keep up with logging my food, paying attention in school, and performing on the track. I unintentionally started losing weight again, and my grades began to slip.

At my lowest, I remember being 118 pounds and feeling terrible. I was tired all the time, didn't want to hang out with my friends, and all I did was run, do homework, eat, and sleep. It was a really sad time of my life. I remember my district cross-country meet, which I had looked forward to all season. I was petrified to race because I was afraid if I stepped on a rock wrong or in a hole, my shin would break. That's how weak I felt. The worst part is, I ended up racing, and winning by a lot. When viewed from the outside, my life at the time looked great. I was the district champ and had individually qualified for the state meet for the first time in my life. This was just weeks before I went into my coma from being too low in sodium. Clearly, even though all my meals may have appeared "perfectly balanced" by numerical standards, they were far from it. I was missing the big picture by a long shot. This is why food restriction can be such a dangerous thing in the sports world, because it is often unintentionally reinforced by coaches and family when it causes your performances to temporarily improve.

## FUELING FOR RECOVERY

One of the reasons many adhere to and become fans of this diet is its ability to help one lower their body fat percentage and "lean out," just as I did during that initial phase. This may be great for the bodybuilding world, but that decrease can be detrimental to high-performing athletes. Without the necessary muscle mass to support activity, athletes are more susceptible to injury (Agel et al. 2007). When I asked if Payton had experienced something similar, she said that two years ago whenever she weighed less, she actually tore her quad. She admitted to me: "I really think it was because I didn't have the lean muscle mass to support my power for sprinting." Not only could improper muscle strength due to inadequate fueling have caused her injury, Payton now knows just how imperative proper fuel is during this period.

She shared that during her healing process, she regrets being too focused on not gaining weight rather than on fueling adequately to help her recovery. She admitted, "When you're injured, sometimes you get scared. You don't want to put on ten pounds and then get back to the track and get hurt again because of the stress the extra weight is putting on your bones. This is the mindset I had at the time, so I ate way less. I was still eating food, but it was not nearly enough. Now if I were to get hurt again, I would make sure that I am taking in the right amount of protein and meeting my caloric needs so that I can hold on to every bit of muscle mass as possible from before my injury. I just take nutrition more seriously now than I did." In fact, Payton was onto something. Studies have shown if calorie restriction is too severe during this time of recovery, muscle protein synthesis needed to repair the injured area and wound healing will slow, and the rate of muscle loss may increase (Tipton 2015; Mettler, Mitchell, and Timpson 2010).

On top of this, the trauma period after an injury or surgery can greatly increase the energy needs of an athlete.

Depending on severity and type, calorie needs may be anywhere from 15–50 percent higher in the beginning phase of recovery (Tipton 2015), and actions like using crutches can take two to three times more energy than walking (Waters, Campbell, and Perry 1987). Clearly, calorie, protein, and micronutrient needs will ebb and flow during this time period, so it is crucial that you not only make sure you are getting proper balance in your meals, but also honoring your hunger cues and listening to your body. Furthermore, this change in diet and decrease in exercise may lead to changes in your physique. It is important to understand this is okay, and even necessary for your body to be able to heal properly and for you to be able to return to the athlete you were before. Just like your training, your dietary needs will go through phases, and if you don't honor the rest periods, your body may not have the built-up energy to sustain the hard training blocks during peak season.

Payton was able to take all these experiences, poor experiences with various fad diets, and knowledge with tracking macros to learn how to eat optimally for her. She shared that she tracked heavily for the first couple months, but then once she got the hang of how to properly build her meals, she stopped. She told me, "Some days I'll go in [to the app] just to see if I'm sticking to it, but it's really taught me how to eat food and how to plan when to eat food to perform at my best."

### BUILDING YOUR OPTIMAL PLATE
All of this to say that meeting one's macronutrient needs can be a game changer, and achieving this doesn't require diligently logging your macros every day. My favorite example of how to

figure out what ratio works best for your training plan is the "athletes' plate" poster that all sports dietitians have. There are essentially three plates for easy, moderate, and intense training days. All of them will contain protein, carbohydrates, and color (fruits and vegetables). Healthy fats should be included as well to help with nutrient absorption and flavor.

The amount of each will vary depending on the day. On an off or easy day, carbs and protein both fill ¼ of the plate and color fills the remaining half. Moderate or in season days will have protein, color, and carbs each filling 1/3 of the plate. Lastly, on hard workout or game days, half of the plate is carbohydrates for quick energy and the other half is split equally between protein and color. As this recommends, there are large differences in our carbohydrate needs depending on the training day, and this is just one of the details that tracking your food in an online platform is not able to currently support.

You may be working out in the morning or at night, and which meals need to be more carbohydrate-dense differ depending on that timing. That is why these basic graphics really do provide such a good base to understand how to build a balanced plate. And if you're skeptical about trusting these plates are actually what you need, don't worry: you are not alone. After tracking my macros for the year prior and thinking I knew everything upon arriving at college, when I saw the "high-intensity" plate half full with carbs, I disregarded it. "That's way too many carbs at one time," I thought to myself. The irony in this memory is rich because that ended up being the main area my diet was largely lacking for that entire year.

Once I met with my team dietitian at Duke, he realized I was eating roughly 200g of protein each day due to my five smaller "perfectly balanced" meals. He shared that this was putting extra stress on my body when I was eating protein where my body was craving carbohydrates. Because I was in such need of energy at this point, my body was having to turn this excess protein into carbs to fuel my workouts, a concept called gluconeogenesis (Adeva-Andany et al. 2016). This left me tired all the time, and unable to perform and train in the way that I knew I could. Now, I often find myself making that very plate with "so many" carbs, so that I can quickly replenish what I burned that day and be equally ready to push my body again in the morning.

All in all, tracking your macros is not necessary as long as you understand what they are and how to balance them at every meal. This is what both Payton and I are now able to do, and you can as well without having to struggle through trial and error like we did. Simply remember those three plate templates and top them with a healthy fat, and you will cover all your important bases customized to your activity needs for that day. Plus, there's so much room for creativity. Whether you have a fresh pesto pasta dinner to fuel a morning race or pack a quick turkey and avocado sandwich with fruit to eat between classes, this skill is one that will be both delicious, and serve you for the rest of your life.

# PAYTON'S FAVORITE WHITE CHICKEN CHILI

For this chapter's recipe, I asked Payton to share her favorite macro balanced meal that she loves to make to fuel her training. She didn't disappoint with this white chicken chili; it is equipped with both beans for sustenance and chicken for a great source of protein. She shared, "This recipe is perfect when the weather turns from summer to fall. Cozy up on the back porch to a bowl of white chicken chili while you root for your favorite college football team. In total, it creates 4 servings of 2 cups each, for a macro breakdown of 29g carbs, 34g protein, and 12g fat."

To make sure you reach your carbohydrate needs for heavy training days, you can serve over a bed of rice or use a fresh, warm bread roll for dipping. Even adding some fresh cheese on top can help add more fat and protein for increased satiation and nutrient absorption! However you customize it, this recipe provides a great base to have a well-balanced and nutritious meal that supports any phase of your training.

*Macros are calculated without the added toppings or sides

**Number of servings:** 4
**Prep time:** 15 minutes
**Cook time:** 35 minutes

**Ingredients:**
- 4 cups of chicken broth
- 3 cups of shredded chicken

- 1 15oz can of cannellini beans
- 2 cans of chopped green chilis
- 1 can of white corn, drained
- 1 onion, diced
- 1 lime, juiced
- 1 tbsp of extra virgin olive oil
- 1 jalapeno, diced (optional)
- 2 garlic cloves, peeled and minced
- 2 tsp cumin
- 1 tsp chili powder
- ¼ tsp of garlic powder
- ½ tsp salt
- ½ tsp pepper
- 1 ranch seasoning packet

**Directions:**

1. In a medium saucepan, sauté onion, garlic, and jalapeno with olive oil. Sauté until slightly softened. Add to the stock pot.
2. Add chicken stock, chicken, beans, green chilis, lime, white corn and all the seasonings.
3. Let all the ingredients cook together for up to twenty minutes or until boiling. The longer it cooks the better it tastes allowing all the flavors to come together.

Garnish with cilantro, avocado, sour cream, fresh shredded pepper jack cheese, and more salt and pepper to your taste preference! The soup tastes even better the next day or can be put in the freezer for up to three months.

## CHAPTER 6

# Aim for a B+

---

*"Remember that sports nutrition principles*
*serve as a guidebook, not a rulebook. It's*
*meant to fuel performance and should*
*never take away from normal life."*

—MEGAN MEDRANO, RD, LD

## EARLY NOVEMBER, 1999

Stanford Sophomore Jesse Thomas did his normal pre-race warm up, took a final swig of water, and toed the line. A hush fell over the crowd as the official raised his hand. "On your mark!" he shouted. "*Pow!*" The gun fired, and 200 of the fastest young men in the United States were off in a blur of tank tops and split shorts. "I knew that all I had to do was have a decent race, and I would make the top seven squad that gets to run at NCAAs," Jesse later explained in his interview with me. It was a ten-kilometer race, and he battled for the majority of the course to be in a good position at the finish.

With about three quarters of a mile to go, he found himself about the fourth or fifth highest placed guy on his team. *All he had to do was finish.*

"And I just faded hard," he recalled. When I asked what was going through his mind at that moment, I could tell it was a clip he had replayed countless times in his head over the years: "I just remember feeling like I was out of gas. I had no energy left. I had pushed my body too far. It was like this little microcosm for four or five minutes of guy after guy running past me—a sort of tangible way to see the cost of how I was trying to achieve my goals."

At this point, you're well equipped with education on how to assess your nutritional needs as an athlete and the importance of not letting outside pressures affect what you put on your plate, but how do you determine when to focus on eating well and when to focus on treating yourself? This is a topic close to the heart of Jesse Thomas, a now-Stanford track alumnus and multi-time Ironman champion who struggled with controlling restrictive eating behaviors during his collegiate career. After years of frustrating moments like this race stemming from his "perfect eating" mentality, he shared with me that he was ultimately able to reach his peak performance and see the most success when he released the reins nutritionally. When I asked him what his main recommendation was for young athletes trying to find their optimal balance, his advice was this: **Aim for a B+.**

## WHERE IT ALL BEGAN

Jesse is a one-of-a-kind athlete. After becoming an NCAA All-American and breaking the school record at Stanford in the steeplechase, he went into the triathlon world and became a twice-over Ironman champion. All three of those accolades are ones people can work their entire lives to achieve, but they were just one part of Jesse's life: his hard work also translated to the classroom and business world. After graduating from Stanford with a major in mechanical engineering, he went on to get his MBA from the University of Oregon and co-found a (delicious) whole foods energy bar start-up called Picky Bars. These bars were some of the first to be sold without highly processed vegetable oils or odd sources of sugars—perfect for a market largely filled with elite athletes. These athletes needed quick fuel for competing that didn't upset their stomachs like the mainstream snacks on the market at that time.

Clearly, he is passionate about sport and nutrition, and has seen much success because of the value he places on using high quality food to fuel his dreams, but he hasn't always had such a balanced plate. In high school, Jesse's nutrition was no better than a typical teenager. Though he was a key player on the basketball, track, and cross-country teams, it wasn't due to his healthy diet as he was largely fueled by pizza and cookies. Once he saw some success and realized he would be able to run collegiately, he realized he couldn't continue with these habits. He told me he became big on the "more is better all the time mentality" and any way that he could "improve" his diet, he did. "From a caloric and nutritional side, it was that everything needed to be cleaner, with no deviations."

This continued for a few years. He dropped his times and felt clear benefits in his fitness from cutting out the fast food and sweets. "It worked for a while," he admitted, but continued, "and then when I got into my sophomore and junior year in college, I started to crack." His biggest goal that second year was to be one of the seven guys representing Stanford at the NCAA national championships. In cross-country, each team races seven athletes and the top five score points based on where they finish: first place scores one point, second scores two, etc. There were so many talented guys on the roster that year that several were fighting for the final sixth and seventh spots, among which was Jesse. No matter who they sent, they would be in the mix for winning a title. It would be an unforgettable experience win or lose, and Jesse knew that.

Rather than let his goal drive him in a healthy way though, he let it consume him. Wherever he could exert control, he did: he trained hard and restricted harder, becoming so obsessed with his eating that he became anorexic. Throughout the entire fall season, he continued this pattern of unhealthy training and lost a significant amount of weight along the way. Unfortunately, it seemed to help; upon arrival at the last meet before nationals that would determine the final roster, he was nearly guaranteed that seventh spot. But his fickle shortcut to success ultimately left him weak and unable to achieve the one goal he set out to accomplish. This all-important meet is the scene he so painfully depicted above. Later that week, his coach let him know he would be traveling to nationals as the eighth man and wouldn't be putting on a uniform to race. He was heartbroken and said that this led to an even less stable relationship with his food where he became bulimic, binging and purging trying to maintain his low "race weight."

As is evident from Jesse's experience, what begins as an innocent intention to compete better can quickly evolve into an unhealthy, and even life-threatening relationship with food. Professional athletes like Jesse are beginning to share their stories and struggles they've had while trying to fuel their intense lifestyles more and more. This openness and vulnerability could be potentially life changing for countless athletes who are trying to push themselves to be the best they can be and might just go about it in the wrong way.

## PUSHING THE EDGE

So, what is the "right way"? This is a hard concept to nail down that even the most objective definitions seem to miss. For example, "health food" is explained on Dictionary. com as "any natural food popularly believed to promote or sustain good health, as by containing vital nutrients, being grown without the use of pesticides, or having a low sodium or fat content." This definition finishes with a great example of how our society can portray only certain foods to be healthy and miss a key concept of balance. As you know by now, nutrients like fat and sodium are crucial to not only our performance as athletes, but our overall health and wellbeing as well. Moreover, as popular media has become more health-conscious, there are more "free" recipes than ever before: dairy-free, sugar-free, gluten-free. If you can name it, it probably exists. Though these can surely be better for us in some ways, the elimination culture they promote can lead to unhealthy fixation on a "perfect" diet, which can evolve into more serious eating disorders like Jesse's.

A 1999 study by Johnson and colleagues found that among college athletes, 35 percent of women and 10 percent of men were at risk for anorexia nervosa, and 58 percent of women and 38 percent of men were at risk for bulimia nervosa (Johnson, Powers, and Dick 1999). This topic is never easy to discuss, and in many cases, these statistics are much higher than reported, but numbers like these prove that it is a prevalent issue within the world of sports, and a risk that all athletes striving for excellence should be aware of. The gray area where a healthy desire to eat better becomes dangerous is already hard to diagnose, but even more difficult for athletes who are often rewarded for keeping a commitment to eating well to better their performance. One of the first studies analyzing this relationship found a high frequency of orthorexia tendencies in both male (30 percent) and female (28 percent) professional athletes across several sports (Segura-Garcia et al. 2012).

So how can you determine if you or someone you know is struggling with this? Where is the line drawn? Libby Lyons, Certified Eating Disorder Specialist (CEDS), shares in an online article that those struggling with this disordered eating "become socially isolated due to their constant planning around food. They may be constantly thinking about food, planning meals or snacks and often lose the natural ability to gauge hunger and fullness... Many individuals struggle to hold 'normal' conversations with others and feel their thoughts become overcome with food. They may experience loneliness, isolation, and think their life has little meaning outside of food" (Lyons 2018).

Elise Cranny, twelve-time NCAA All-American and Olympian in the 5000m, vouched for how a controlling relationship with her diet had spillover consequences on other avenues of her life. In a podcast with *Voice in Sport*, she shared of this experience during her freshman year of college: "I was pretty heavily restricting my eating... It was detrimental to my training and performance, but also mental health, happiness, and life in general. When your body and your brain aren't getting what you need, it's really hard to focus in school. You're just more irritable. You are just more unhappy in general" (Cranny 2020). As she shares in this vulnerable quote, these behaviors can be life-impeding. Even when she was able to push past sacrificing her personal happiness, Elise described how after scrutinizing over everything she ate all day, she wasn't left with any energy to mentally be at her best when competing, describing it as not having that "extra edge" when the race gets hard. She is now a huge advocate of eating healthy fats and a whole foods diet rather than attempting to restrict food to cut time by losing weight. Incredible success has resulted from her new habits, such as being a part of the world record holding 4x1500-meter relay, setting the American record in the indoor 5k, and representing America in the Olympics.

**YOUR WORDS MATTER**

All of this to say, no one is immune from going down this unhealthy path, and what you say to others matters tremendously. Even just a side comment can turn into a cue that launches someone down this slippery slope, so being aware of the prevalence of these issues is extremely important.

When speaking with Jesse about where he began to see his thoughts like this develop, he took me back to when his cross-country team was at training camp in Mammoth Lakes, CA. There, he and his teammates were running anywhere from eighty to over one hundred miles a week at nearly eight thousand feet of elevation and were, as he put it, "just burning calories like crazy." You can imagine how difficult this training is. If fueling isn't taken seriously in these extreme conditions, injuries can occur quickly and often, but that wasn't what the young boys were concerned about. Jesse remembers a twisted common afternoon joke when a teammate would say, "Oh, I'm really hungry, I'm gonna go take a nap." This comment clearly perpetuated underlying misconceptions that lighter is faster and is a great example of how innocent comments or jokes can be harmful. There's no telling what the young freshman thought when the teammates they were looking up to promoted unhealthy habits like this.

As I write this, I am sitting on the couch in Crested Butte, Colorado, training at the highest level I ever have in my entire life (literally and metaphorically). I am at nine-thousand-foot elevation myself, running sixty miles and lifting three times per week, and the most confident with food and running that I ever have been. Just last night, I went out to dinner with my parents and some family friends and much to everyone's surprise—ordered a burger with fries. I find it funny how many questions people ask about my "diet" when they learn that I am passionate about nutrition. In this particular situation, I was asked if it was my "cheat day" because I ordered a burger. Thankfully, I was in a place where I knew what a proper plate looked like for me that night, but for someone struggling with letting themselves eat "normal" food, the comment could have been extremely unnerving.

My confidence came from an awareness of the big picture of my diet and a clear understanding of how that burger fit perfectly into it. My workout that morning was thirteen miles, and the beef was from a local farm. This burger bun was rich with carbs to replenish my energy reserves, the beef high in iron, protein, and fat to help my blood carry more oxygen and nourish my muscles back to health after a hard day of training. This wasn't a cheat meal; it was actually a perfectly balanced plate for what my body needed at that moment. To be clear, I'm not saying you need to run thirteen miles to have a burger. My point is there is a way to live a healthy lifestyle that includes enjoying the foods you love, and it is important to remember that food shouldn't carry "good" or "bad" labels. Make an effort to allow yourself these moments to relax and reframe the way you think about what is and isn't "healthy" for you. This is what Jesse was able to do after going to such an extreme trying to be part of that top seven on his team at Stanford.

## FINDING THE BALANCE

Jesse took this painful time in his life and rather than giving up because of it, learned from it. Once he realized what he was doing wasn't sustainable, he began to educate himself and learned how to fuel correctly, became a badass *and* well-fed athlete, and used his experience to help others realize they don't have to go through the same mistakes as he did. He has become adamant about spreading awareness that male athletes are just as susceptible to disordered eating behaviors as their female counterparts and encouraging younger guys as well to be proactive about avoiding these unhealthy beliefs: "The way that I look at it, male athletes should be seeking out nutrition advice in the same way they seek out coaching or weightlifting advice. In fact, it's a core pillar of athletic performance. It's not even a question of avoiding a potential eating disorder problem so much as maximizing your performance as an athlete, and that's the way men and women really should look at it."

As soon as I heard him mention that his philosophy was to aim for a B+, I knew this would have to be the title of its own chapter. As someone who has come a long way to figure out herself that this is the best philosophy to live by, I hope I can help it resonate with you enough to pursue your healthy lifestyle with whole foods and lots of cooking, but also the occasional guilt-free treat.

Jesse admits, "It took me nearly two years from that point to understand that I was going to eventually find my peak athletic performance—better than I was when I was a sophomore at the very tip of the obsessive compulsive drive by finding balance and developing this nutritional philosophy that was to aim for a B+. What I eat is mostly healthy, but I know that if I go for an A, it's going to crack me." Learning this lesson in his early twenties as a runner is undoubtedly what helped him to reach such success in his professional career as a triathlete. Now he is a father to two happy and healthy children and mentions that he and his wife keep the terminology "bad" and "good" foods away from both their company at Picky Bars and their home. He lets himself enjoy his favorite yogurt covered pretzels and lucky charms, and lets his children enjoy them too, along with many home-cooked and nourishing meals that bring them just as much happiness.

Maddie Alm, the Olympic trials qualifier in the 5k and registered dietitian whom I interviewed earlier in the book, gave a great example of this in one of her Instagram posts. I vividly remember scrolling through my feed one day and seeing her story where she posted a bowl of sugary cereal that she was having. Her caption was about how there can be points in time when yes, even the snack your mom never let you eat, can be great for an athlete. Whether it is for replenishing carb stores or even just quenching a sweet tooth craving—it doesn't matter. When I saw that an expert in the area of nutrition was enjoying one of the most notorious "unhealthy" foods, it made me so happy. Not only because I am an avid cereal lover (my grandma calls me "her cereal girl"), but also because I know so many young athletes felt relief upon reading that a professional athlete and dietitian had this sweet breakfast option on her approved menu.

## THE EXPERT ADVICE

It is important not to overlook that yes, body composition can have an effect with athletic performance, but it may not be exactly what you have in mind. Jesse shared that he has absolutely seen benefits from being a bit leaner for peak competition season, but he was clear that there exists a healthy way to get your body to its best state, and working with a registered dietitian can be key in finding that place: "There were parts of my career where I was able to find that balance, and then there were parts where it was way off. And what sounds like a core pillar to your book is that balance exists in different ways depending on who you are. The most important thing you can do is speak to a professional because every person and every body is unique." As you pursue pushing your body to its peak performance, understanding what a healthy balance looks like is extremely important. Megan Medrano, RD, LD, describes three characteristics of a well-balanced athlete from her website Run Whole Nutrition:

1. They stay flexible - preparation allows them to not get anxious about food at social events, and easily be able to adapt when the food plan doesn't turn out exactly as they thought it would.

2. Food morality does not exist - you're not "better" than anyone else because you eat healthier, and you certainly don't deserve to "punish" yourself after indulging in a cookie or some M&Ms.

3. They listen to their bodies - when they are craving something salty, they listen and eat some pretzels, and they are well in tune with and respect their hunger cues.

She shares this further in an article she wrote titled "When Healthy Eating Goes Too Far: The Link Between Orthorexia and Athletes," where she adds, "When an athlete has a flexible, intuitive, and thoughtful approach toward nutrition, they view it as an *ally*. They use principles of sports nutrition to guide their eating decisions, while also cultivating interoceptive awareness and attunement to determine the most appropriate choice at that moment"(Moderno 2019). If you keep the motto of aim for a B+ when choosing your fuel, it will allow you to do exactly that. When you aren't stressing about joining your teammates for ice cream because you know you have had healthy nourishing meals all day long, it un-demonizes these treats. This freedom allows you to better listen to and distinguish when your body and soul could really benefit from an Oreo shake, versus when you actually aren't that hungry and would rather just go along for the company.

## YOU ARE NOT ALONE

Whether it is Jesse's, Elise's, or my experiences that resonate with you the most, they all have something in common: we are sharing them. What I hope more than anything as you're learning how to build your own B+ diet, is that you find others around you to bounce your ideas off of and learn with. What the proper diet looks like for you as an athlete, and how to best avoid developing unhealthy relationships with food, are not topics that should be taboo to talk about! Learning your best fueling plan is an ever-evolving process and one that is always beneficial to bounce off other people when you aren't sure if your plate is correctly balanced. Jesse mentioned how important surrounding yourself with a group that embodies a supportive culture of having healthy conversations about food and fueling is, especially with the people that you spend every day with like your teammates and coaches. Everyone else has to go through the same process of figuring out what balance looks like for them, and this journey can be hard and isolating if you have to navigate it alone.

Where a professional can give you advice on where your nutrients are lacking, your peers can provide a sounding board and emotional support in a different way because they understand your life on a much deeper level. Additionally, eating is an aspect of your life that will never go away, and something that is constantly on all our minds, so making the environment one where people feel comfortable bringing up their concerns can alleviate an incredible amount of social pressure and be extremely beneficial for everyone involved. Not only can you potentially gain insight from those around you about how they have approached similar struggles, sharing these intimate experiences will bring you closer together and give you a bond that could potentially help you compete better on the field or court. Thus, if you can find and surround yourself with people who you feel comfortable talking about these hard topics with and are confident they will always answer with your best interest as a person, not just an athlete, in mind, you are already in a great spot. It is important to note you don't have to put pressure on yourself for all your relationships to be this perfect source of support either, as that is unrealistic. You already know what to do. Just aim for a B+.

# QUINOA CRUST MARGHERITA PIZZA

This gluten-free and high-protein pizza is super easy and delicious and will help you get whole foods while still enjoying an indulgent classic. With that being said, this is also a reminder that if you want the real deal, I fully support you in that endeavor as well. This has been my favorite go-to meal to make for my family when staying in Colorado at altitude because of its versatility and ability to please the pickiest of pallets. I will give you ideas for how to top it, but my main focus here will be the dough, which is super simple and made from just quinoa, avocado oil, chicken broth, and seasonings. All you have to do is blend them together and pour on a baking sheet for a whole foods and delicious crust that is just as tasty as the real thing. Here I added simple toppings for a margherita style cheese pizza, but feel free to add any others that you may desire. P.S. You may have to double the recipe, as it tends to disappear quickly!

**Number of servings:** 2
**Prep time:** 10 minutes
**Cook time:** 30 minutes

**Ingredients:**
- 1 cup quinoa
- ½ cup chicken broth
- 1 tablespoon avocado oil
- 1 tablespoon garlic and herb seasoning
- 1 teaspoon smoked paprika
- 1 ½ teaspoons salt

- ¾ cup no sugar added pasta sauce
- 2 cups shaved parmesan
- 1 tomato
- 1 package or 6–8 fresh basil leaves
- No stick baking spray (avocado oil preferred)

## Directions:

1. Soak the quinoa in a bowl with 1 cup of water for 60 minutes.
2. When the quinoa has about 5 minutes left to soak, preheat the oven to 375 degrees Fahrenheit, and line a baking sheet with foil. Make sure to spray the foil with your non-stick spray
3. Rinse off your tomato and basil and cut them both into very thin slices.
4. Once the quinoa is finished soaking, drain out the excess water and scoop into a blender along with the avocado oil, chicken broth, and seasonings.
5. Blend until you get a thick paste, and pour out onto the sprayed foil
6. Bake the crust for 14 minutes, making sure to leave the oven on when it finishes
7. Once this is finished and the crust hardens, remove the pizza, and spread on the pasta sauce, making sure to leave the edges bare if you like a crunchy crust. Then, spread the 2 cups of parmesan evenly on top of the sauce
8. With the new toppings, return the pizza to the oven and bake for 5 more minutes at 375 degrees.
9. Then, remove the newly warmed dish and add your final garnishes: the thinly sliced tomato and fresh basil leaves. If desired, you can also add precooked meat

or vegetables at this stage. I personally love to add another final sprinkle of parmesan on top.

10. Return to the oven and set it to broil. Let it cook for 3 minutes, while watching carefully. This browns the cheese and crust, so you can broil a little longer if you prefer a crispier bite.

11. Remove from the oven and cut into slices. Devour.

## CHAPTER 7

# Social Sugar

———

*"If you want to go fast, go alone. If
you want to go far, go together."*

—UNKNOWN

**LATE APRIL, 2005**

On one particularly hot summer day after roughly twenty
hours of traveling, Allen Lim arrived in Girona, Spain, hungry, tired, and irritable. As one of Spain's culinary hotbeds,
the promise of Girona's authentic Spanish cuisine was the
one thing that had gotten Allen through his exhaustive journey. He set his bags down in front of the apartment and
mustered up the energy to knock. Footsteps echoed through
the crack under the door which finally swung open to reveal
Floyd Landis, American cyclist and 2006 champion of the
Tour de France. Allen had finally arrived.

After getting moved in, Allen imagined he and Floyd would
head out to a local restaurant and indulge. Then, with their

bodies well fueled and primed for sleep, they would return home and get the rest he had been looking forward to all day. But the renowned cyclist had a different idea. He took one look at Allen, and immediately remarked, "Whoa, you look like crap. Are you hungry? Do you want to eat?"

Allen responded with an enthusiastic, "Hell yeah. Where are we gonna go?" But rather than answering, Floyd welcomed him in and went straight to the kitchen. He grabbed the milk from the fridge, opened up the cupboard, and started pouring a bowl of Lucky Charms for his famished guest. It was precisely at this moment that Allen realized he was in trouble. He thought to himself, "If this is how we're gonna try to win the Tour De France, it is not gonna happen." That night, Allen took Floyd to the local supermarket, and thus began his long-term endeavor to help change the way the cycling community approached fueling from the ground up.

Since that day in Spain, Lim has gone on to serve as a consultant for the Chinese and United States Olympic teams, written three cookbooks on athletic nutrition, and founded a sports fueling company, Skratch Labs. One may not normally think a Doctorate in Exercise Physiology would extend to the kitchen, but as we've seen from prior chapters, the two are intimately connected. Even as a thirteen-year-old, Allen had already recognized this underappreciated connection between the two worlds. He grew up in the Philippines with a burning passion for cycling and two genuine "foodies" for parents. After watching them make home-cooked meals, young Allen, a clear entrepreneur, ended up spending countless hours in the kitchen finding ways to create his own fuel to sustain him during rides. Just like the now widely used "gel packs" by endurance athletes, he would bite off the corner of a Ziploc bag he had filled with canned peaches and honey to use as fuel when on his home-grown Tour de France. That warm night in Girona, he realized that he would get to combine this passion for fueling he discovered so young with his work training elite athletes and has gone on to do so in an incredible manner.

## UNDERSTANDING THE PRO CYCLING WORLD

I first knew of Allen from my own experience using some of his company Skratch Labs' hydration mixes to fuel longer workouts. Because of his focus on natural ingredients, different sugars, and a meticulously calculated carbohydrate to electrolyte ratio, it never upsets my stomach and has powered me through the workouts that I feel most proud of. Upon starting my interview with him for this book, I thought he would talk mainly about hydration or making sure to consume high quality foods in your meals. I had no idea of the insight he would bring to me with regards to the immense psychological impact eating with others can have on your performance as well.

For those who aren't familiar with the details of pro cycling, athletes competing in the Tour de France, a.k.a. "Le Tour" or "Le Grande Boucle," compete in twenty-one different stages, one each day, with each taking about five and a half hours to complete. Across the twenty-one days and over 2,100 miles, the average 150-pound rider will burn anywhere from 5,000 to 8,000 calories a day. It is hard to conceptualize just how much food this is to consume, so imagine a meal containing a three-egg omelet, two slices of toast with either butter or jelly, and a piece of fruit, roughly 600 calories. That means these athletes could potentially have that meal *ten times* (thirty eggs) and *still* be in a caloric deficit. Obviously, that is unrealistic, and many of the athletes have several packs of gels, bars, and sports drinks during their ride to help sustain their carbohydrate reserves throughout the event.

Once they finish competing for the day though, it is imperative that they fulfill the rest of their caloric needs with nutrient-dense foods in order to repair all the damage and stress they have put their body through. *This* is why it was so concerning to Allen when Floyd pulled out Lucky Charms as if it were a completely normal dinner. "Despite the fact that I was an exercise physiologist, and I was there to design training programs, if I didn't help these kids to eat right, it wasn't going to matter," Dr. Lim realized. He had been hired to work for Floyd, Lance Armstrong's then-best friend and famously talented American cyclist. Allen knew others expected a lot from him and that getting his athletes to eat well could really set them apart from their competitors.

After Allen's realization that the cycling world needed a food upgrade, he began to spearhead many homemade staples to keep the athletes well fueled. He helped to build food trucks and hire professional chefs who made everything from scratch and slowly started teaching the athletes how to eat properly, to fuel their intense levels of training. What's more, this new aspect of training wasn't just an effort to benefit the athletes' health; it was also a direct effort to combat the rampant doping that was clouding the sport at the time.

## IF YOU TAKE SHORTCUTS, YOU GET CUT SHORT

Floyd Landis went on to become the 2006 winner of the Tour de France, but his title was ultimately revoked after a positive doping test result from that year. On top of needing to help turn around the way the cycling world fueled, Allen was essentially thrown right into the midst of the largest performance enhancing drug (PEDs) scandal in sports. This was a rude awakening for someone who grew up with posters of professional cyclists lining his walls and looked up to the athletes at this level of sport his whole life. He told me, "As a cycling fan, I hoped, like most fans, that the cyclists I admired were clean... My naive optimism, however, was shattered. Ultimately, that trauma gave me the motivation and courage to work to make a difference—to make sure that the hell of that period of time would never be an option for the next generation of riders and staff."

Doping is defined by *Merriam-Webster* as "the use of a substance (such as an anabolic steroid or erythropoietin) or technique (such as blood doping) to illegally improve athletic performance," and boy was there a lot of it in the cycling world at that time. When talking about this struggle with me, Allen stated, "I think that the meals were a way to give athletes an alternative that was better than all of the performance enhancing drugs that were being used." Notice that Dr. Lim says "meals" here, not food or micronutrients. One of the largest discoveries he has had over his time working with elite athletes both nutritionally and physically is the importance of these athletes sharing their meals with people who support them. Although the dependence on steroids or PEDs is extreme, many professional athletes can also turn to viewing their nutrition as their "edge" in the same way and become anal about measuring each morsel of food that they consume.

Their hope is that this micro-managing of food will help them stay leaner and make sure they don't over or under fuel. What people don't think about though, when they first start to calculate calories or macros, is the joy that it takes out of both the food itself and the action of eating with others. Allen saw this time and time again through his work with athletes competing at the elite level and knew he had found something big. When talking about the potential he believed his discovery could have, he stated, "I got into this because I realized that **there was a social component to food that was potentially equally as performance enhancing**" as the drugs being used.

## SOCIAL SUGAR

Thus, the main message of Dr. Lim's 2016 cookbook *Feed Zone Table* encourages athletes to never eat alone. He discusses how for society as a whole, the ethnocentric approach to food is slowly disappearing as we get more focused on our personal goals and become "too busy" to share a meal with others. To do so would require planning a time to meet, prepping food, and actually carving out sixty to ninety minutes to eat with others while having conversation—a wholly inefficient way to consume food you could easily have eaten in about twenty minutes alone! This is exacerbated for athletes who, whether due to travel, training, or being tired, naturally spend a lot of time solo. This dilemma combined with the fact that elite athletes tend to have a much higher rate of eating disorders (ED) than the general population (Sundgot - Borgen and

Torstveit 2004), substantiates the connection between loneliness and ED's (Levine 2012). When eating alone, it's easy to get wrapped up in an unhealthy mindset with food because there is nobody else there to keep you accountable. Prevalent stereotypes of what athletes in your sport "should" look like can become overpowering when there aren't people next to you as a reminder that they love you exactly how you are.

What Allen's and his co-author Biju K Thomas' research reveals is that the physiological effects of loneliness will hinder one's performance more than a fast-food hamburger ever could. The palpable effects this feeling can have on one's health were exposed by a 2020 study by the National Academies of Sciences, Engineering, and Medicine. In this paper, it was found that social isolation and loneliness were associated with a 29 percent increase in one's risk of heart disease and a 32 percent increased risk of a stroke (Donovan and Blazer 2020). Hence, it is no surprise that if loneliness affects your heart health this significantly, it could hinder your physical performance as well.

As Allen puts it beautifully, "During my own time spent coaching athletes in Europe, I discovered firsthand that nothing could bolster or limit performance as much as one's mental wellbeing. A simple dinner with great company could inspire the power to win, while something as seemingly common as loneliness could be the loose thread that, when pulled, unraveled everything." Whether this tendency to eat alone develops from wanting to eat at a different time, avoiding the gaze of others, or because they want particular ingredients and proportions, what starts as "just one meal" can quickly spiral into the norm.

Jason Donald, a former pro cyclist and All-American runner, wrote the preface in Lim's book where he adamantly agreed with the importance of this simple action. He states, "Being a pro comes with benefits, the kind we talk about, but the sheer force of that drive to be faster can be isolating... When I eat a meal with people I love, the experience meets a deep-seated need that goes well beyond my body's need for carbohydrates, protein, and fat" (Lim and Thomas 2015).

This is powerful coming from someone who has spent ten-plus years in sport and has seen the way his body reacts to all types of stimuli, whether nutritional or social. It's almost as if the online list of superfoods should include "any food eaten with the people who love and care for you," because of the benefits this can have to our overall mental and physical health. Sports can drive people into a rat race of seeking external approval, working alone for months on end to achieve a goal, and then as soon as they have it, the shiny medal gets old and the process starts all over again. Those athletes who constantly incorporate this new type of super food into their lives—let's call it **social sugar**—are able to avoid burnout by finding their value in the people they love and that love them, rather than taking on the immense stress and pressure that comes from finding self-worth through their performances. Allen said it best in *Feed Zone Table:*

**"If there's anything we have learned from sport and life, it's our happiness and health that drive performance and success, not our performance or success that makes us happy or healthy."**

## MY EXPERIENCE

As an athlete at Duke, I have felt this firsthand. One time specifically, I remember even bringing my laptop into the athlete dining area, grabbing my plate of chicken, rice, and a salad, and finding a seat alone at a corner table so that I could finish grinding out a long reading that I had to have done for my class at eight the next morning. I'm not sure where I got the idea that I would be able to eat and focus at the same time, let alone in a room with 200 other athletes, but I did not feel like losing track of time chatting at dinner only to arrive home and still have four hours of work to do.

After three of my teammates all individually stopped by to see why I was alone and how my day was, I realized something: I had spent thirty minutes in the dining hall putting up a strong facade of being a multitasking queen yet had gotten absolutely nothing done. At that moment, I took a deep breath, shut my laptop, packed up my stuff, and went to sit next to my roommate at the dinner table. Immediately, I was welcomed with jokes about my attempt to do work and questions about my day and knew that I had made the right decision. I left that dinner feeling more energized and happy than I had in over a month, and was ultimately able to think more clearly and finish my reading faster than if I had just droned right on through dinner.

As you grow older and even become a collegiate or professional athlete, it will only get more difficult to find time to eat with others as training, recovery, or school begin to take more and more of your time. *But the crazier the schedule gets, the more important it becomes to take the time to sit down for a meal with others.* It can be overwhelming to have a burning drive and desire to eat well, use whole foods and healthy oils, and get the recommended amount of micronutrients, yet also want to go out with your friends, or appreciate the box cupcakes made by a teammate. I'm not saying you absolutely must eat the fried chicken your family got for dinner, but I encourage you to make an effort to take part in meals with the people in your life.

One way I love to approach scenarios where I know I won't want to eat the food, is to fuel well beforehand and then make a small plate at the event. I can take a couple of bites here and there, but I mainly go for conversation and bonding time. This often allows me to still feel good about the food that I ate without making the hosts or those at the event feel like I don't want to eat what they provided. Everyone's situations will be different depending on your cultural norms and your personal food preferences, dietary needs, or restrictions; you may feel comfortable bringing your own food, or not making a plate at all. The right way will always be the one that makes you feel the most comfortable and still connected with those around you.

If you are so focused on fueling your muscles and body perfectly that you are depriving your soul from the nourishment that spending time with others can provide, you'll never be able to truly enjoy and be present for the moments you worked so hard for. However, you choose to take these words to heart, whether it's routine pancakes at your apartment after a long run, or going to a Mexican restaurant after an all-day soccer tournament, I promise you won't regret it. Cherish these moments with your team. Not only will it help you all to compete better and be happier, but it will also help create memories and relationships that last a lifetime.

# FREAKY FAST STEAK FRIED RICE
(Can swap protein if desired!)

This recipe is one of my favorite meals I have ever made for my team because of the raving reviews it received. It is super easy to throw together in thirty minutes and double or triple to serve a crowd of any size! Not only will you be getting in your social sugar, but this meal is also actually sneakily full of protein, veggies, and probiotics for the ultimate recovery meal after a long day. The beef is easily substituted for chicken or tofu to make it perfect for your needs—it is a small portion anyway because it's mostly added for the flavor. The meal is already protein rich from the edamame and eggs! On heavier workout days you can always add more rice, or if it's an off day you can sub a cup of cauliflower rice if you want! For all the veggies, I prefer to buy mine pre-chopped and frozen because it saves so much time that is usually worth the extra dollar or two. Don't delay: text your teammates and tell them to come over to help you whip up this delicious dish and enjoy it together.

**Number of servings:** 3
**Prep time:** 10 minutes
**Cook time:** 25 minutes

**Ingredients:**
- ½ cup chopped onion
- 3 cups cooked rice
- 1 cup peas & carrots (if frozen, thaw before use)
- 1 cup edamame (extra protein)

- 4 tbsp avocado oil (the safest oil for cooking at high temperatures because of its high smoke point)
- 2 chopped green onions
- 6 eggs
- 1 cup cooked ground beef (or chicken, turkey, or tofu)
- seasoning of choice (I love Montreal steak seasoning and Mrs. Dash garlic and herb)
- ½ cup soy sauce (use gluten free if desired)
- 1 tbsp mellow white miso paste (great source of probiotics for increased gut health)

**Directions:**
1. Warm the avocado oil in a LARGE pan on heat and add in the 1/2 cup chopped onion.
2. Put your eggs in a bowl to scramble them while you wait and save them for a later step! You can add a bit of milk if desired to make them fluffier.
3. Once the onion begins to caramelize, throw in your peas, carrots, edamame, green onions. Even if they're frozen, that's okay. In that case just throw them in a bit earlier.
4. Add your scrambled eggs into the pan and stir every 30 seconds or so.
5. Once the eggs are just about done, turn the heat to high and add in your pre-cooked protein and rice.
6. While your delicious creation warms in the pan, add your soy sauce and miso paste to a small bowl and whisk in the miso to make a perfect Asian fusion sauce for your rice.
7. Once warm enough (after about 5 minutes), put your fried rice in a large serving dish and let your guests pour the sauce over their meals as desired. Heat can kill the probiotics in the miso paste, so it's better to let the rice cool a bit before adding!

## CHAPTER 8

# No More Sand Foundations

———

*"You cannot build a dream on a foundation of sand.*
*To weather the test of storms, it must be cemented*
*in the heart with uncompromising conviction."*

—T.F. HODGE

### JULY 6, 2016

Sunlight glimmers off of a strong and beautiful naked body hovering in the air. A volleyball floats in the forefront, about to be crushed by the posed athlete. Stark tan lines decorate her back. The intensity is palpable. Standing at 6'1 and holding herself with such an air of confidence and preciseness, it is clear that this is not the first time she has gone through this motion. The camera snaps. The athlete falls back down to the trampoline, which she was jumping on to pose for the dramatic shot.

This is one of the most powerful images from *ESPN Body* magazine, both artistically and literally. The star was three-time Olympic medalist April Ross. Featured in the 2016 edition alongside Dwayne Wade and Antonio Brown, April's photos highlight both her physical prowess and her comfort in her own skin. Though that may seem logical, as she is at the pinnacle of her sport, athletic success does not always correlate with increased body confidence. In fact, when athletes are propelled into the public eye, this glory often comes with a detriment to their mental health from being judged on every aspect about them.

## FUELING FOR PERFORMANCE VS. FUELING FOR AESTHETICS

In her interview that accompanied the vulnerable *ESPN* piece, April spoke about how she has seen this pressure play out in her sport: "Sometimes the idea of a beach volleyball body gets mixed up with the casual beach goer, lay-out-in-a-bikini type. For me, I value the power of my body, and I think I'm a little more muscular than you might expect. I don't consider myself thin, and I'm not trying to look great in a bikini—I'm trying to be as strong as possible and as powerful as possible for my sport." This quote is just one of many that demonstrate what an incredible role model and person April is. Young girls now have someone sharing at an early age that they don't need to let outside pressures influence their nutritional choices and relationships with their bodies. She is helping countless athletes leave the sand on the volleyball court, rather than use it as a weak foundation for the incredibly important trio of nutrition, body image, and self-confidence.

Though she is an expert now, April once had to figure out how to combat these thoughts herself. "I was definitely self-conscious about my body for the first couple of seasons out on the beach. I was always focused on positive self-talk for myself," she admitted, but added that this positive self-talk wouldn't have held any weight without her making solid nutritional choices to back up her confidence in her fitness: "If I was content having the positive self-talk but just eating pizza and drinking soda all day, that's obviously not going to be as effective as me sacrificing eating that crap and trying to eat healthier year after year. Feeling the difference and even seeing the difference, that's going to work a lot more."

In other words, the confidence and belief she developed in her body and its ability to carry her to an Olympic gold medal was reinforced by the nutritious meals and snacks that she fueled with, not a shining six pack. Though physical changes can certainly accompany a healthier diet, she puts her focus on how her food will help her feel more sustained on the court and allow her body to reach its maximum capability. April is a great example of how finding this love for the body you have can both help you reach your peak performance and be a star in the world's top athlete magazine.

**THE RESEARCH**
More and more athletes are speaking about this pressure they feel from social media and society to look a certain way. There isn't just one type of athlete who is susceptible—even the most seemingly "fit" people feel pressure to improve their bodies in some way. Kate Grace, US Olympian and Nike track athlete, shared in a blog titled "Race Weight" that: "A running

career has added body image pressure… Sponsorships involve racing in skimpy uniforms, as well as photoshoots and other sports modeling. While it's billed as empowering, and it can be, it didn't feel that way during that period. I more than once burst into tears from the idea of having photos taken; I was so uncomfortable in my skin" (Grace 2019). This makes my heart ache as a runner who looks up to Kate and all her amazing accomplishments, especially thinking about all the mental strain it caused. Just as April has the pressure of competing in a bikini, the professional track race kits have a similar style sports bra and underwear appearance, and the effects of these pieces of clothing are evident.

For example, research comparing a control group of noncompetitive women to female athletes in "leanness sports" such as running revealed that the percentage of those who had experienced eating disorders greatly increased for the elite female athletes, 7 percent as opposed to 21 percent in the control group (Torstveit, Rosenvinge, and Sungdot-Borgen 2007). It is so easy for the comparison game to begin in these situations and for unhealthy patterns to develop before you even really notice it. Disordered eating and a broken relationship with one's body and food can inhibit both one's personal life and performance and are hard to recover from. Women in strength sports have their own battles as well, where they feel a strong sense of conflict when the same strong muscles that help them excel in their sport don't conform to the societal image of what it means to be "feminine" (Petrie et al. 2002). This can be seen in our media anywhere you look. Whether it's a Twitter troll saying tennis legend Serena Williams is "built like a man" or a 2021 *New York Times* article written by Matthew Futterman that received backlash after saying skier Jessie Diggins "looks like a sprite in her racing suit," the judgment on athletes and their bodies is ever present.

Are the uniforms reinforcing this unhealthy relationship with food? In an article for team USA titled "Why Do Some Athletes Struggle with Body Image?" clinical psychologist Melissa Streno explained that "when you think about perfectionism and orderliness and compulsivity, that predisposes some of these athletes to be rigid about the way they look in their uniforms, what they eat, and how much they work out in order to influence their body image." Corroborating research from 2012 found that revealing uniforms not only negatively affect female volleyball players' body image but can also directly hinder their performances (Steinfeldt et al. 2012). Having examples like April and Kate who are proud of their muscular bodies and are willing to share about their struggles is invaluable. They are helping young athletes realize the beauty in their strength and ultimately avoid years of mental and nutritional struggle.

What I'd like you to focus on, though, is the inverse: The positive effect a strong body image can have on your success. A 2019 study on NCAA Division 1 athletes found a clear association between athletes' positive body image and their sport confidence and flow state. I'm sure most of you have felt it, but flow state is essentially when you are 100 percent focused in the moment of the game or match, seem to lose your perception of time, and are able to perform at extremely high levels. The researchers reasoned that this correlation could be due to better body image allowing for more focused attention on the task at hand and therefore greater chances of one's ability to achieve this prime state (Soulliard et al. 2019).

Moreover, this is among people who were confident enough to compete in the first place; another study on high school and college students found that there was a significant correlation between self-esteem and sports participation (Ouyang et al. 2020). In other words, how people view themselves can keep them from both participating in sports *and* being able to compete to their best ability. For an attribute that is seemingly out of our control and hard to measure, this can be scary to think about. Just imagine how many potential Olympians and professional athletes didn't even start a sport because they were never able to get past this stage. That is why the example that April sets is so important, and why I want to share her journey to reaching this level of confidence and ability.

### WHERE IT ALL BEGAN

Seventh-grade April didn't have quite the same swagger on the court as she does now. Though she loved volleyball immediately, she recalled to me how she didn't make the cut for her team that year. Like Marshall though, she is not one to take no for an answer. She went on to letter in three sports at Newport Harbor High and was awarded Gatorade National Player of the year in volleyball. When I asked her how she fueled during such a great time of growth and accomplishment in high school, she revealed that her parents did an incredible job of providing nutritious meals throughout: "My parents had a big garden in their backyard and my mom cooked really healthily, so I never had to worry about it. It wasn't until way after that I realized how healthy we ate." In an environment where the food was homegrown and fresh off the stove, she was able to both thoroughly enjoy her meals and feel the benefits of such food on the court. As great as this was, it didn't mean that she understood what was helping her succeed, or how to continue this healthy relationship with food once she got into college.

Just as I'm sure many of you have heard about or experienced yourself, April's college of University of Southern California provided a dining hall just for athletes called *training table*. We have the same thing here at Duke, and it's pretty much exactly what you would imagine. For us at least, you walk in to be hit with the aroma of fresh pasta and roasted vegetables alongside a weak but striking aroma of sweat and dirt from the athletes who come straight from practice (guilty). The circular tables span the wide space and aside from the occasional cross team friend group breaking all the norms, everyone is typically seated with their respective teammates. The food is self-serve, and you can walk up and scoop up as much as you want of any of the four meal options for that day and, if you're sneaky, take home leftovers in a to-go container. A typical day would provide me the choice between some chicken, green beans, and rice combo, freshly made pasta, salmon and roasted sweet potatoes, or a delicious sushi bowl garnished with edamame and seaweed salad. Clearly, there is plenty of choice, and with the dessert section being equally decadent, the options can be overwhelming.

When April shared with me about her experience in a similar situation, she said, "The way I viewed it, this is the food they're giving to athletes, so it must be healthy, and I can eat as much as I want here. I just had no one guiding me in the right direction. So like a lot of people, I gained the freshman fifteen, and then spent the rest of my college career trying to lose it and figure out how to eat properly." April found what many of you have already realized: learning how to grasp the ideal combination of quality, quantity, and timing of what fuel works best for you is a constant learning process. She was adamant that the issue wasn't that she gained weight, it was that she did so without knowing what she needed and when. In many cases, an athlete may gain healthy weight when learning how to fuel properly, as this can be part of the learning process.

Again, fueling for performance is not the same as fueling for aesthetics. If you have slowed down training, you might lose a little "leanness", and that is okay. As long as you are eating balanced nutritious meals and listening to your hunger cues, your body will fluctuate and go through changes throughout your season. In order to be able to stay healthy and fit through your intense competition seasons, you must let your body relax when you do get time off. Trying to fight these changes and maintain a certain physique or exact weight year-round will not only be nearly impossible but can also have serious negative effects on both your mental and physical health. Just like April, you will encounter new environments and new food choices, and have to read just what works best for you all the time. All I ask is that you remember that the body that you feel the worst in and the one that you perform the best in are *the same one*. It is the most consistent thing in your life, and it is extremely important that you love it throughout all of its phases.

## GUYS, I'M TALKING TO YOU TOO

Whether you're an athlete on the track, a male swimmer in a speedo, or a beach volleyball star like April, this pressure is ubiquitous among the sports world. Erin Rubenking, associate director and clinical care coordinator for the University of Colorado Athletic Department's Psychological Health and Performance program, is outspoken on this stereotype, remarking, "There is a misconception that eating disorders are disorders for females. The reality is that men struggle with eating disorders just like women do… It often takes men a much longer time to get help because of that" (Burtka 2019).

As you saw in a previous chapter with Jesse Thomas, all athletes can feel the pressure to be thin, but there is an equally detrimental effect from the opposite pressure of needing to appear "bigger." The official term is called *muscle dysmorphia,* where one is trying to alter their body to achieve a certain ideal physique, specifically a desire to be more muscular. Muscle dysmorphia is considered a type of body dysmorphia when the individual believes something is wrong with their body. Sometimes athletes may interpret themselves as small when in fact they are very muscular and become obsessed with looking at their muscles in the mirror, known as *body monitoring.* Studies documenting athlete responses noted that these individuals have reported that their concern with their nutrition schedule and gym plan interfered moderately with their life, that they spend at least three hours a day thinking about needing to become muscular, and some avoid people and places due to their concerns about their body (Tod, Edwards, Cranswick 2016). Rebecca Youngs, MS, RD, LD, stated, "This type of body dysmorphia is more common in males, but it is still prevalent in females, particularly those in sports like bodybuilding. It may just present and be experienced differently for these women."

Several male athletes have come out to speak on the issue as well. The Indianapolis Colts' offensive linemen made an appearance in the 2015 *ESPN Body Issue* where they shared about their struggles in the sports world. One of the three interviewees, Anthony Castonzo, admitted that "in middle school, I used to refuse to play basketball shirtless outside because I was afraid people would see me and I was not happy with my body. Then when I was in high school, I thought, 'Oh, I'm too skinny, I need to put more muscle on.'" His perceptions of how people would judge his body inhibited him from playing as much as he wanted to growing up. Maybe he would have become a professional basketball player rather than a football player if not for this feeling; there's no way to tell.

Through this experience though, he has gathered great insight and touched on how taking care of one's self-image is an ongoing process: "I don't think a perfect body is attainable. Even giant bodybuilders who are super muscular may not have the flexibility or athleticism that someone who's smaller has." Clearly, the pressure to look a certain way isn't limited to the beach volleyball court or female athletes like April. In fact, there are sports where these pressures are literally embedded in the rules like wrestling and boxing, or the scoring is subjective like gymnastics and figure skating. In studies examining the participation of NCAA athletes in weight control behaviors, up to 85 percent reported participating in either self-induced vomiting, excessive exercise, and/or the use of weight loss supplements (Chatterton and Petrie 2013; Clifford and Blyth 2018; Power et al. 2020).

When you break down your foundation like this, everything else begins to fall with it. On top of the physical and mental health detriments that accompany these actions, they can carry over to cause poor athletic and academic performance (Joy, Kussman, and Nattiv 2016). Whatever your sport or background, there will always be someone else who is "faster" or looks "fitter" at some stage, and it is important that you always remember to keep your eyes on your own journey so that you don't fall into this trap. Focus on how your differences make you unique and give you an advantage, rather than viewing them as something holding you back from reaching your goals.

One person who is a great example of taking charge of this is Olympic gold and bronze medalist Cody Miller. Cody was born with a congenital deformity where his sternum grows inward, so the middle of his chest is caved in. It's easy to see how this can be hard to deal with as not only an athlete, but as a swimmer who spends 90 percent of their time practicing and competing shirtless. As a high schooler, he recalls going up to the blocks in a t-shirt every time, and not feeling fully at ease until he hit the water. So what helped him go from quaking on the blocks to winning arguably the most coveted athletic award? It ended up being therapy.

After beginning his sessions to work through some familial problems, he ended up being able to release years of thoughts and self-doubt about his appearance. He shared in an interview with Jeff Burtka, "For the first time in my life, I actually really opened up and talked about it, and it helped. It 100 percent helped. It helped make me feel more confident." He continues by noting that "when you have those internal feelings, it doesn't get better until you let it out... It didn't take winning a gold medal for me to love myself or appreciate the way that I looked. It was just recognizing that there's nothing wrong with looking a little different" (Burtka 2019). This is just one example of many that demonstrates how significantly the way athlete's view their bodies can affect their mental health and therefore, their athletic performance. Because Cody is an extreme case in both his condition and his success, he should undoubtedly serve as an inspiration to talk to someone if you need help finding confidence in the power of your body.

## THE PATH TO SUCCESS

So how did April emerge from college and become the incredibly confident and successful woman she is today? I asked her, expecting her answer would reveal her turnaround sometime while in school, but she shared that this was not the case. "It wasn't until Team USA provided a registered dietitian for us and I started playing at the highest level that I started to dial in my nutrition. I think it's one thing I really could have used at a younger age, especially in college." After years of packing brown paper bag lunches and guessing at what she thought was the best fuel for her performance, she learned how much more room she still had to grow in making sure the meals she made herself were actually giving her what she needed.

If you're someone who doesn't like cooking—April is with you. She shared, "Eating healthy has to be super simple and easy for me; I don't really do anything that requires a recipe." Every Sunday afternoon before dinner, she does her weekly grocery shop and meal-preps for the week. "I definitely have to schedule it in and be dialed in. Otherwise, there's like no chance I'm doing it." Her willingness to try new things and figure out what works best for her schedule and needs combined with working with a registered dietitian has helped her find balance and incredible success even though she had a very late start.

She told me she has experimented a lot with her nutrition, but the one thing she has always stuck by is making sure she is eating enough. "There's a lot of calorie restriction in my sport, and I've always tried to fight against that and make sure I'm eating enough," she shared. "Even if throughout the years that means I'm five pounds heavier than someone else of my size, I know it's allowed me to maintain my energy and endurance longer." When I asked her if she had a particular role model she studied to find this nutritional confidence, she replied, "I've never really followed anybody nutritionally; I've just talked to experts and listened to my own body to figure out what works best." After having to teach herself nutrition for years, and experimenting with veganism, vegetarianism, and paleo diets, she has finally reached a place where she feels confident with her fuel just being composed of nutritious, homemade meals.

## THREE ACTIONS TO INCREASE BODY CONFIDENCE

1. Make a list of all the amazing things your body has accomplished

   This can seem frivolous, but it can be powerful. It will allow you to reflect on all your body has done for you so far and realize its wild untapped capability for when you have confidence and trust in your fuel.

2. Find a role model in your sport that has a similar body type to you

Make sure to read their comments on the topic and confirm they are someone who has a healthy food and body image relationship. If they have come out and spoken about this publicly already that would be ideal. Then if you'd like to reach out, they are much more likely to be willing to talk to you about their experiences and give you tips relevant to your sport!

3. Never be afraid to talk to an expert

As you have seen from both Cody and April, speaking to experts like sports psychologists and registered dietitians can be pivotal in helping you build the trust and security in your fuel that will help you reach your athletic goals.

## LOVE YOUR BODY

First and foremost, what is important is that you realize just how incredible your body is. Even on an off day, your body is constantly working, breaking down food, sending blood to your brain, and storing your precious memories for you to be able to live a long and fulfilled life.

Accepting and loving your body "as is" is easier said than done, but the work will be worth it once you begin to feel the positive effect it has on both your self-confidence and performance. No matter what gender, weight, sex, or race you are, you should never feel as though you have to change to look like the "ideal athlete" for your sport.

Whoever is reading this, I hope we can be the change and start reminding ourselves and younger athletes not to play this dangerous comparison game. It is important that you take these steps *now* to care for your relationship with your body *before* it becomes an issue. The ultimate goal: that you are always making balanced nutritional choices according to what will make you *feel* the best, rather than *look* the best. With this knowledge, you'll be able to stop trying to appease others' expectations of how you should fuel and look, and divert your energy toward becoming the best athlete you can possibly be.

# PEANUT BUTTER BANANA PROTEIN PANCAKES

This delicious and protein-packed crowd pleaser is my favorite recipe of them all. I have made them countless times for family and seen them topped with everything from maple syrup and fresh banana slices to a fried egg. I think the savory pancake route is so underrated. On top of this, the easy-to-make batter can be thrown in a waffle maker as well! All you have to do is throw the ingredients in a blender before baking into your desired shape, and you'll be able to appease the hungry crowd in no time. Enjoy these pancakes knowing they will help you begin to build this foundation of strong confidence in your fuel and performance, as the ingredients are all specially picked to help recover and replenish your body for training the next day.

**Number of servings:** 4
**Prep time:** 5 minutes
**Cook time:** 10 minutes

**Ingredients:**
- 3 eggs
- 3 bananas
- 2 1/4 cup oats
- 2 tsp baking powder
- 1 tbsp cinnamon
- 2 tsp vanilla
- 1 1/2 cups almond milk (can sub if desired)

- 3/4 cup peanut butter powder
- 1 tsp salt
- No stick baking spray (avocado oil preferred)

**Directions:**
1. Throw all ingredients in a large high-speed blender, and blend until you have an evenly mixed batter.
2. Warm a pan on medium heat, and spray with the avocado oil so that the pancakes don't stick.
3. Pour the batter into the pan in your desired pancake sizes, and sprinkle in any additional ingredients you may want to make your perfect pancake (chocolate chips, cocoa nibs, coconut flakes, sliced banana).
4. Cooking times will differ depending on the thickness of your pancakes, but a good check is to flip them once you begin to see little bubbles.
5. After flipping, let them cook for about 30 more seconds or until both sides are a golden brown.
6. Stack as high as you'd like and personalize to your heart's desire! You can never go wrong with the classic maple syrup dip or layering on a fried egg. Call me crazy, but I like to do both!

## CONCLUSION

# The Bell Lap

———

*"Nothing in life is worthwhile unless you take risks. Fall forward. Every failed experiment is one step closer to success."*

—DENZEL WASHINGTON

Writing *The Players' Plate* has been a labor of love for which I will be forever grateful. When the world was turned on its head during the COVID-19 outbreak, writing gave me purpose. I decided to create something that would last forever and that people could immediately recognize as a tool in fueling their athletic dreams. Originally, I had a basic title that tied together the concept of athletes and sports nutrition, but as I neared the end of writing the book, I realized a key concept that every athlete I had interviewed touched on was not encompassed in that title ... the importance of balance. Thus, *The Player's Plate* was born. This metaphor, symbolizing the importance of us finding balance both on our plates and in our lives, just fit perfectly. What I didn't realize would be the equally invaluable, yet more subtle lesson encompassed within it. One that I had to learn myself the hard way even throughout the process of writing this book: **the importance of being open to change**.

During my freshman year at Duke, I had just begun feeling like I was making friends in my new home of Durham, North Carolina, and my first fall collegiate cross-country season was behind me. I was excited for outdoor track in the spring, where the 3,000-meter steeplechase was going to be my main event. We were supposed to hold the ACC Conference Championship on our home track. I had my sights set high. With 35 cement barriers (hurdles) and 7 water pits spread throughout the 7.5 lap race, this was a lively event that allowed me to utilize both my height at 5'8 and my multisport athleticism gained through years of volleyball and basketball.

Interestingly, a year earlier during my senior year of high school, when I realized that was the event I would be focusing on at Duke, I looked up the 2020 Olympic Trials qualifying time: 9:48. Though I had just recovered from a coma and was totally new to the event, I set all my passwords to 0948. Yes, I know I'm going to have to pick a new one now. If there was one thing that I thought about daily to motivate me to stick to a consistent bedtime and prioritize eating high quality meals, it was that time. Now a year removed from those high school dreams, I was about to get to see how lofty they actually were. I packed a small suitcase to go home for spring break, already excited to return.

Then, one quick phone call changed everything. "Have you seen the news?" my teammate asked. After seeing that all schools had been shut down for the rest of the year, including

Duke, I realized it would have to be another *year* before I could chase this dream I had been working so hard toward. Everything we had taken for granted and thought of as normal disappeared before our eyes. Classes went online, sports came to a complete stop, and families lost loved ones. For the next four months, I found myself training back in Houston without even a goodbye to my newfound friends and teammates. This time was extremely tough for me, as I'm sure it was for all of us.

After losing that freshman track season, we weren't guaranteed that we would have a cross-country season the following fall either. Thus, I decided to take a gap semester away from school and competing for Duke. That was when I began writing this book. It was a scary decision to step away from the new friends and routines I had just built, but I didn't want to take classes online, nor blow another season of eligibility. I also knew I would get so much more out of creating this resource that could help so many other athletes, so I decided to go for it. This experience, full of change and adjusting, proved invaluable in helping prepare me for the next big hurdle in my running career. One that I would face the very next year.

We all recognize, and I know I've mentioned in several chapters, how important consuming enough carbohydrates is to reach one's athletic goals. It was something I personally focused on improving as I began my collegiate running career. Despite my efforts, as I undertook my sophomore and junior seasons while writing this book, I was still having trouble translating the progress I was making in practice to competitions. My junior year cross-country season was especially hard. At the fittest I had ever been, I was crushing workouts, but couldn't seem to translate it to race day. I vividly remember lining up for the NCAA Regional Championships. At the halfway point of the 6k race, I was in perfect position within the front pack. That's when I began to see stars. Slowly but surely, I started to fade, and by 1k left, I was barely above a jog. It took all I had just to stay on my feet and not pass out so that I could finish the race. I finished 146th that day and averaged a time that was 30 seconds per mile *slower than my tempo workouts.* It was one of the hardest days of my life.

Nothing made sense. I was the one eating healthy, always going to bed early, and writing a book on sports nutrition. Why couldn't I even run a normal race without nearly blacking out halfway through? I knew something was wrong, so immediately upon returning to campus, I reached out to my team doctor. After a series of conversations and tests, I was ultimately diagnosed with celiac disease. In short, this is when gluten (included in products with wheat, rye, and barley like bread and pasta) causes an autoimmune reaction where your body begins to attack the villa on the inner lining of your small intestine. This causes one to struggle with nutrient absorption from their food. Essentially, I was constantly undernourished because I couldn't absorb many of the key vitamins and minerals that I needed. By doing what I was told would be beneficial for an endurance athlete, eating carbs, I was doing more damage by invoking this inflammatory response in my body. It's ironic considering all the work I had done over the past two years to get myself to eat more bread and pasta.

Thus, I began buying gluten free products and experimenting with this new aspect of my life I had to come to terms with. Celiac disease is different from gluten intolerance. This condition can only be diagnosed by a medical professional via blood test and intestinal biopsy, and the only "cure" is to completely avoid gluten. In fact, you have to be extremely careful about wheat slipping into seasonings and food products that you typically wouldn't expect, because even a crumb can set off a series of negative effects. I did my best to put forth the extra effort to embrace this new lifestyle in the same way that I did when I had my sodium scare. To make that recovery process less daunting, I carried around a giant saltshaker that I affectionately named Sal. Now, I never travel anywhere without my delicious gluten free pretzels. It can be hard to find gluten free foods that are also carbohydrate rich at restaurants, like rice and potatoes, so I am constantly planning ahead to make sure I can meet my needs without inconveniencing anyone around me. From my sodium scare to this diagnosis, if there's one lesson that I have learned, it is that one's journey with nutrition is an ever-evolving process.

Though those years and experiences have been extremely difficult, this final and most recent discovery has been life changing for me. As I entered my junior year spring outdoor track season, exactly two years since COVID shut down my freshman year, I really began to feel like myself when running again. It reminded me of how good I felt that final year of high school when I fell in love with the sport in the first place. All the dots began to connect. When looking back, I realized that during that final stretch of high school when I changed my diet dramatically, I was unintentionally eating gluten free. More recently, even though breads and pastas were not a huge part of my everyday diet, I always made sure to eat them in order to carb load before race days. I didn't realize that was why my body was so unwell every time I stepped on a start line.

It was like someone had handed me the final piece to a puzzle that I had been trying to finish my whole life. I finally realized exactly what *my body* needed to thrive. When I lined up for that junior year ACC Outdoor Championship meet on my home track… the one that we were supposed to host two years prior, I knew it was going to be a special day. How special though, I could never have imagined. The previous year, my best time in the steeplechase had been a 10:25. Throughout my junior season, I lowered this to a 10:15, and had my eyes set on breaking that 10-minute barrier and placing myself within the top 5 all-time at Duke. On that warm night in North Carolina under the Friday Night Lights, I ran a 9:48.

Nearly a 30-second PR and the school record, it was the biggest breakthrough of my running career. The time earned me a silver medal and All-ACC honors. A couple weeks later, I also earned a ticket to race in the NCAA Championships at the famous Hayward Field in Eugene, Oregon. There, I earned my first All-American honor. And this was just the beginning: my conference time also qualified me for the USA Outdoor Track & Field Championships which would equate to the Olympic Trials during Olympic years. Here, I raced against Olympians, national champions and other professional runners that I had been watching on TV for years and finished #16 in the USA. It all felt like a dream.

I will be forever grateful for how authoring this book during the past couple of years undoubtedly helped me reach these goals. Just as it helped me feel grounded in a world turned upside down by the pandemic, working on the final edits two years later allowed me to keep my mind occupied between the workouts and long travel days of this incredibly exciting time. There was so much changing in my life and *The Player's Plate* provided a constant. Writing it has been just as beneficial to me as I hope reading it has been for you. By following the advice of all the athletes about balance and finding what plate worked best for *me* (which was gluten free), I was able to become the runner I had always dreamed of being.

Clearly, it took a long time for me to finally reach this place, and I realize I still have a long way to go. My journey of figuring out what nutrition strategies work best for me has been far from linear. Naturally, your journey will be full of the same highs and lows along the way, but I hope that if I can be an example of one thing, it's that they will all be worth it. Whether your main takeaway from the lessons the athletes I interviewed and I share focuses on building a balanced plate, getting better sleep, or sharing more meals with loved ones, I am looking forward to seeing all that you can accomplish with this head start.

The biggest challenge with putting all this information into a static book, though, is that I can't update it. I did my best to make the concepts as basic and fundamental as possible, but inevitably, there will be studies that come out after this publication that provide new perspectives. Each time new discoveries in the world of sports nutrition are made, both your view and the literature on nutrition can and will evolve.

That is perfectly normal. In fact, it's necessary. Understand that this is going to be a part of your journey and always keep an open mind so that you never stop learning along the way. This may be my final chapter, but your story is just beginning. If you are able to get comfortable embracing change, there's no telling how many of your crazy dreams might just become a reality.

# Acknowledgments

First and foremost, I'd like to thank Eric Koester and the Creator Institute for creating a program where I could make this book a reality.

To Megan Hennessey and Colin Lyon, my editors and biggest cheerleaders, I would never have made it to the finish line without your constant help and support. Thank you for believing in me even when my faith wavered.

To my mom and dad, DaNae and Stephen, I wouldn't be anywhere near where I am today without your unwavering love and support. I am well aware of how lucky I am, and I thank God every day for y'all.

To my sisters Julia and Kristin, thank you for setting the bar so high and being such incredible examples for me to follow in life. And to my new brother-in-law Martin, thank you for reminding me to be proud of myself. Forever grateful for you all. Love you infinity! #Coleteam

To my beta readers who provided a new perspective and helped me rethink what my true vision for *The Players' Plate* was, thank you. My entire family above, plus Bex, Dan, Matt, and Melia, you were all an incremental part of this journey as well.

To all my teammates, coaches, and friends for all the constant support in my journey, even when I missed out on events to "turn in a chapter" or "work on revisions," thank you for always being there for me.

To all the athletes and experts I interviewed, thank you for vulnerability and insight. This book wouldn't be the same without your incredible stories.

Special shoutout to my dear friend Rebecca Youngs. Bex, you served as a beta reader, professional reviewer, and confidant all in one. Thank you for coming in like the fourth quarter MVP and shoving me to the finish line. Words can't express how grateful I am for you.

And last but certainly not least, thank you to everyone who pre-ordered this book what seems like so long ago, and supporting me and my author journey since the very beginning:

Delyssa DeClue, LaDonna Johnson, Kristin Cole, Sondos Moursy, Keri Smith, Jim Garrison, Allison Rand, JJ Foster, Payton Chadwick, Judy Parsons, Emmie Bultemeier, Alyson Freeman, Eric Koester, Julia Cole, Imee Villarreal, Taylor Morrow, Lizzy Davidson, Natasja Beijen, Sydney Casey, Adrianna Tedford, Staci Fleming, Chris Frezza, Scott Mayo, Presley Miles, Rhonda Riley, Julie Fitzpatrick, Claire

McConnell, Libra Thompson, Sam Caillouet, Laura Smith, Jack Smith, Nancy K. Westfall, Lance McRae, Nadine Ndip, Angela McRae, Timothy McGuire, Marjorie Locker, Katrina Pena, Laura Nunziata, Kelly K. Flavin, Sara Stephenson, Connor Erlandson, Lauren Caillouet, Colleen Zajicek, Naima Turbes, Michaela Reinhart, Leigha Torino, Ruby Duncan, Alex Nguyen, Joshua Karas, Lauren Rocco, Robert McGee, Cameron Andrews, Curtis Ward, Virginia Blackwell, Paul Johnson, Nancy Gregory, Darryl Langley, Kathlene Francis, Sandra Belcher, Catherine White, Camyar Nazari, Kevin Firebaugh, Bo Martinovich, Annie (Besson) Briscoe, Adele Caillouet, Drew Wagner, Tony Della Fiora, Renee Ballard, Joel Smith, Kami Knake, Stephanie Beard, Courtney Locke, Grace Boudreau, Gabrielle Richichi, Kirsten Handler, Georgia Stavrinides, Paula D Cole, Zach Barry, Genaro Villar, Jackson Flash, Kim Frost, John Ghetti, Will Dixon, Christopher Theodore, Angie & Judd Kaiser, Morganne Gagne, Abby Pickett, Nina Ferreyra, Kristen Veit, Rory Cavan, Elizabeth Reneau, Francesca Cetta, Cameron Tharp, Mike Ungvarsky, Sherry Bowersock, Kaili Rasberry, Peter Sterzing, Michael Breiter, Jack Kovach, Charlotte Tomkinson, Emily Sauer, Chuck Cannon, Lacy West, Landry Lemoine, Sherrie Sherertz, Grace Fenter, Antonia Anderson, Elena Meyers, Dean Rios, Josh Romine, Jeff Craig, Jonathan Boyda, Aziz Hatamleh, Kaz Kasowski, Aaron Black, Sarah Scalia, Jordan Bar, Jarrett Reyes, Julia Harter, Matthew Fecteau, Olivia Hennig, Emily Harvard, Kedaar Sridhar, Breanna Lipscomb, Sheila Moeller, Veronique Koch, Ann Knoyle, Valerie Bachmann, Allison Slovak, Theo Burba, Mike Thibodeaux, Joe Robertson, Mike Mclaughlin, Kameron Barrera, Austin Shockley, Brithany Coss, Michael Greene, Laura Baustian, Nick Wilson, and Melody Grady

# Appendix

---

**INTRO**

Christensen, Natalie, Irene van Woerden, Nicki L. Aubuchon-End-sley, Pamela Fleckenstein, Janette Olsen, and Cynthia Blanton. "Diet Quality and Mental Health Status among Division 1 Female Collegiate Athletes during the COVID-19 Pandemic." *International Journal of Environmental Research and Public Health* 18, no.24(2021): 133-77. https://doi.org/10.3390/ijerph182413377.

Matsuoka, Shiho, Miyuki Tsuchihashi-Makaya, Takahiro Kayane, Michiyo Yamada, Rumi Wakabayashi, Naoko P. Kato, and Miyuki Yazawa. "Health Literacy Is Independently Associated with Self-Care Behavior in Patients with Heart Failure." *Patient Education and Counseling* 99, no. 6 (2016): 1026–32. https://doi.org/10.1016/j.pec.2016.01.003.

Meegan, Amy, Ivan Perry, and Catherine Phillips. "The Association between Dietary Quality and Dietary Guideline Adherence with Mental Health Outcomes in Adults: A Cross-Sectional

Analysis." *Nutrients* 9, no. 3 (2017): 238. https://doi.org/10.3390/nu9030238.

Torres-McGehee, Toni M., Kelly L. Pritchett, Deborah Zippel, Dawn M. Minton, Adam Cellamare, and Mike Sibilia. "Sports Nutrition Knowledge among Collegiate Athletes, Coaches, Athletic Trainers, and Strength and Conditioning Specialists." *Journal of Athletic Training* 47, no. 2 (2012): 205–11. https://doi.org/10.4085/1062-6050-47.2.205.

Webber, Kelly, Stoess, Amanda, Forsythe, Hazel, Kurzyneske, Janet, Vaught, Joy Ann, and Bailey Adams. Diet Quality of Collegiate Athletes. College Student Journal, 49, no. 2 (2015): 251-256. https://eric.ed.gov/?id=EJ1095696.

## CHP. 1

Avena, Nicole M., Pedro Rada, and Bartley G. Hoebel. 2008. "Evidence for Sugar Addiction: Behavioral and Neurochemical Effects of Intermittent, Excessive Sugar Intake." *Neuroscience & Biobehavioral Reviews* 32, no. 1 (2008): 20–39. https://doi.org/10.1016/j.neubiorev.2007.04.019.

Freeman, Clara, Amna Zehra, Veronica Rameriz, Corinde Wiers, Nora Volkow, and Gene-Jack Wang. "Impact of Sugar on the Body Brain and Behavior." *Frontiers in Bioscience* 23, no. 12 (2018): 2255–66. https://doi.org/10.2741/4704.

Friesen, Carol, Kilee Kimmel, Kimberli Pike, and Karin Lee. "Annals of Sports Medicine and Research Sports Nutrition Knowledge, Sources of Nutrition Information, and Desired

Sports Nutrition Advice of Collegiate Student- Athletes at a Division I Institution." (2021).

Hull, Michael V., Andrew R. Jagim, Jonathan M. Oliver, Mike Greenwood, Deanna R. Busteed, and Margaret T. Jones. 2016. "Gender Differences and Access to a Sports Dietitian Influence Dietary Habits of Collegiate Athletes." *Journal of the International Society of Sports Nutrition* 13, no. 1 (2016). https://doi.org/10.1186/s12970-016-0149-4.

Jeukendrup, Asker E., Luke Moseley, Gareth I. Mainwaring, Spencer Samuels, Samuel Perry, and Christopher H. Mann. "Exogenous Carbohydrate Oxidation during Ultraendurance Exercise." *Journal of Applied Physiology* 100, no.4 (2006): 1134–41. https://doi.org/10.1152/japplphysiol.00981.2004.

Madero, Magdalena, Julio C. Arriaga, Diana Jalal, Christopher Rivard, Kim McFann, Oscar Pérez-Méndez, Armando Vázquez, et al. The Effect of Two Energy-Restricted Diets, a Low-Fructose Diet versus a Moderate Natural Fructose Diet, on Weight Loss and Metabolic Syndrome Parameters: A Randomized Controlled Trial." *Metabolism* 60, no. 11 (2011): 1551–59. https://doi.org/10.1016/j.metabol.2011.04.001.

Torres-McGehee, Toni M., Kelly L. Pritchett, Deborah Zippel, Dawn M. Minton, Adam Cellamare, and Mike Sibilia. "Sports Nutrition Knowledge among Collegiate Athletes, Coaches, Athletic Trainers, and Strength and Conditioning Specialists." *Journal of Athletic Training* 47, no.2 (2012): 205–11. https://doi.org/10.4085/1062-6050-47.2.205.

## CHP. 2

Asche, Angie (@eleatnutrition) "Have you heard any of these myths about protein? Let's break each one down. Please tag + share with someone who may find this helpful! A common myth people have heard about protein is that [...]." Instagram, June 17, 2021. https://www.instagram.com/p/CQOrQEhAROt/?hl=en.

Barry, Daniel W., Kent C. Hansen, Rachael E. Van Pelt, Michael Witten, Pamela Wolfe, and Wendy M Kohrt "Acute Calcium Ingestion Attenuates Exercise-Induced Disruption of Calcium Homeostasis." *Medicine & Science in Sports & Exercise* 43, no. 4 (2011): 617–23. https://doi.org/10.1249/mss.0b013e3181f79fa8.

Bell, Douglas G., and Tom M. McLellan. "Exercise Endurance 1, 3, and 6 H after Caffeine Ingestion in Caffeine Users and Non-users." *Journal of Applied Physiology* 93, no. (2002): 1227–34. https://doi.org/10.1152/japplphysiol.00187.2002.

Calder, Philip C. "N–3 Polyunsaturated Fatty Acids, Inflammation, and Inflammatory Diseases." *The American Journal of Clinical Nutrition* 83, no. 6 (2006): 1505-1519. https://doi.org/10.1093/ajcn/83.6.1505s.

Cox, A. J., D. B. Pyne, P. U. Saunders, and P. A. Fricker. "Oral Administration of the Probiotic Lactobacillus Fermentum VRI-003 and Mucosal Immunity in Endurance Athletes." *British Journal of Sports Medicine* 44, no. 4 (2008): 222–26. https://doi.org/10.1136/bjsm.2007.044628.

Daley, Cynthia A, Amber Abbott, Patrick S Doyle, Glenn A Nader, and Stephanie Larson. 2010. "A Review of Fatty Acid Profiles and Antioxidant Content in Grass-Fed and Grain-Fed Beef."

*Nutrition Journal* 9, no. 1 (2010). https://doi.org/10.1186/1475-2891-9-10.

Dei Cas, Michele, and Riccardo Ghidoni. "Dietary Curcumin: Correlation between Bioavailability and Health Potential." *Nutrients* 11, no. 9 (2019): 2147. https://doi.org/10.3390/nu11092147.

DePhillipo, Nicholas N., Zachary S. Aman, Mitchell I. Kennedy, J.P. Begley, Gilbert Moatshe, and Robert F. LaPrade. "Efficacy of Vitamin c Supplementation on Collagen Synthesis and Oxidative Stress after Musculoskeletal Injuries: A Systematic Review." *Orthopaedic Journal of Sports Medicine* 6, no. 10 (2018): 232596711880454. https://doi.org/10.1177/2325967118804544.

Environmental Working Group. "Clean Fifteen Conventional Produce with the Least Pesticides." 2019. https://www.ewg.org/foodnews/clean-fifteen.php.

Farrokhyar, Forough, Rasam Tabasinejad, Dyda Dao, Devin Peterson, Olufemi R. Ayeni, Reza Hadioonzadeh, and Mohit Bhandari. "Prevalence of Vitamin D Inadequacy in Athletes: A Systematic-Review and Meta-Analysis." *Sports Medicine (Auckland, N.Z.)* 45, no. 3 (2015): 365–78. https://doi.org/10.1007/s40279-014-0267-6.

Featherstun, Meghann (@featherstonenutrition) "Is that freaking true Friday? Each Friday 1 of your fab nutrition questions answered in T/F form. Collagen is a good protein powder replacement. FALSE. Lots of questions last week led […]." Instagram, May 22, 2020. https://www.instagram.com/p/CAfQNY5nchE/

Gualano, Bruno, Hamilton Roschel, Antonio Herbert Lancha, Charles E. Brightbill, and Eric S. Rawson. "In Sickness and in Health: The Widespread Application of Creatine Supplementation." *Amino Acids* 43, no. 2 (2011): 519–29. https://doi.org/10.1007/s00726-011-1132-7.

Guest, Nanci S., Trisha A. VanDusseldorp, Michael T. Nelson, Jozo Grgic, Brad J. Schoenfeld, Nathaniel D. M. Jenkins, Shawn M. Arent, et al. "International Society of Sports Nutrition Position Stand: Caffeine and Exercise Performance." *Journal of the International Society of Sports Nutrition* 18, no. 1 (2021). https://doi.org/10.1186/s12970-020-00383-4.

Hill, C. A., R. C. Harris, H. J. Kim, B. D. Harris, C. Sale, L. H. Boobis, C. K. Kim, and J. A. Wise. "Influence of β-Alanine Supplementation on Skeletal Muscle Carnosine Concentrations and High Intensity Cycling Capacity." *Amino Acids* 32, no. 2 (2006): 225–33. https://doi.org/10.1007/s00726-006-0364-4.

Hooda, Jagmohan, Ajit Shah, and Li Zhang. "Heme, an Essential Nutrient from Dietary Proteins, Critically Impacts Diverse Physiological and Pathological Processes." *Nutrients* 6, no. 3 (2014): 1080–1102. https://doi.org/10.3390/nu6031080.

Hultman, E., K. Soderlund, J. A. Timmons, G. Cederblad, and P. L. Greenhaff. "Muscle Creatine Loading in Men." *Journal of Applied Physiology* 81, no. 1 (1996): 232–37. https://doi.org/10.1152/jappl.1996.81.1.232.

Jäger, Ralf, Chad M. Kerksick, Bill I. Campbell, Paul J. Cribb, Shawn D. Wells, Tim M. Skwiat, Martin Purpura, et al. "International Society of Sports Nutrition Position Stand: Protein and Exercise." *Journal of the International Society of Sports Nutrition* 14, no. 1 (2017). https://doi.org/10.1186/s12970-017-0177-8.

Khatri, Mishti, Robert J. Naughton, Tom Clifford, Liam D. Harper, and Liam Corr. "The Effects of Collagen Peptide Supplementation on Body Composition, Collagen Synthesis, and Recovery from Joint Injury and Exercise: A Systematic Review." *Amino Acids* 53, no.10 (2021): 1493–1506. https://doi.org/10.1007/s00726-021-03072-x.

Khosla, Sundeep, Merry Jo Oursler, and David G. Monroe. "Estrogen and the Skeleton." *Trends in Endocrinology & Metabolism* 23, no. 11 (2012): 576–81. https://doi.org/10.1016/j.tem.2012.03.008.

Killer, Sophie C., Andrew K. Blannin, and Asker E. Jeukendrup. "No Evidence of Dehydration with Moderate Daily Coffee Intake: A Counterbalanced Cross-over Study in a Free-Living Population." Edited by Dylan Thompson. *PLoS ONE* 9, no. 1 (2014): e84154. https://doi.org/10.1371/journal.pone.0084154.

Kirkpatrick, Kristin. "Should You Pay More for Cage-Free or Organic Eggs?" Health Essentials from Cleveland Clinic. March 18, 2016. https://health.clevelandclinic.org/should-you-pay-extra-for-cage-free-or-organic-eggs/.

Kulczyński, Bartosz, Joanna Kobus-Cisowska, Maciej Taczanowski, Dominik Kmiecik, and Anna Gramza-Michałowska. "The Chemical Composition and Nutritional Value of Chia Seeds— Current State of Knowledge." *Nutrients* 11, no. 6 (2019): 1242. https://doi.org/10.3390/nu11061242.

Li, Haojie, Meir J Stampfer, J. Bruce W Hollis, Lorelei A Mucci, J. Michael Gaziano, David Hunter, Edward L Giovannucci, and Jing Ma."A Prospective Study of Plasma Vitamin D Metabolites, Vitamin D Receptor Polymorphisms, and Prostate Cancer." *PLoS Medicine* 4, no. 3 (2007). https://doi.org/10.1371/journal.pmed.0040103.

Loureiro, Laís Monteiro Rodrigues, Eugênio dos Santos Neto, Guilherme Eckhardt Molina, Angélica Amorim Amato, Sandra Fernandes Arruda, Caio Eduardo Gonçalves Reis, and Teresa Helena Macedo da Costa. "Coffee Increases Post-Exercise Muscle Glycogen Recovery in Endurance Athletes: A Randomized Clinical Trial." *Nutrients* 13, no. 10 (2021): 3335. https://doi.org/10.3390/nu13103335.

Margolis, Lee M., Jillian T. Allen, Adrienne Hatch-McChesney, and Stefan M. Pasiakos. "Coingestion of Carbohydrate and Protein on Muscle Glycogen Synthesis after Exercise: A Meta-Analysis." *Medicine & Science in Sports & Exercise* 53, no. 2 (2020): 384–93. https://doi.org/10.1249/mss.0000000000002476.

Nogoy, Kim Margarette, Bin Sun, Sangeun Shin, Yeonwoo Lee, Xiang Zi Li, Seong Ho Choi, and Sungkwon Park. "Fatty Acid Composition of Grain- and Grass- Fed Beef and Their Nutritional Value and Health Implication." *Food Science of Animal Resources* 42, no. 1 (2022). https://doi.org/10.5851/kosfa.2021.e73.

Nybo, Lars, Peter Rasmussen, and Michael N. Sawka. "Performance in the Heat-Physiological Factors of Importance for Hyperthermia-Induced Fatigue." *Comprehensive Physiology* 4, no. 2 (2014): 657–89. https://doi.org/10.1002/cphy.c130012.

Pedersen, David, Sarah Lessard, Vernon Coffey, Emmanuel Churchley, Andrew Wootton, They Ng, Matthew Watt, John Hawley, and J Hawley. "First Published May 8." *J Appl Physiol* 105 (2008): 7–13.

Pedlar, Charles R., Carlo Brugnara, Georgie Bruinvels, and Richard Burden. "Iron Balance and Iron Supplementation for the Female Athlete: A Practical Approach." *European Journal of Sport Science* 18, no. 2 (2018): 295–305. https://doi.org/10.1080/17461391.2017.1416178.

Perim, Pedro, Felipe Miguel Marticorena, Felipe Ribeiro, Gabriel Barreto, Nathan Gobbi, Chad Kerksick, Eimear Dolan, and Bryan Saunders. "Can the Skeletal Muscle Carnosine Response to Beta-Alanine Supplementation Be Optimized?" *Frontiers in Nutrition* 6 (August 2019). https://doi.org/10.3389/fnut.2019.00135.

Puente Yagüe, Mirian de la, Luis Collado Yurrita, Maria J. Ciudad Cabañas, and Marioa A. Cuadrado Cenzual. 2020. "Role of Vitamin D in Athletes and Their Performance: Current Concepts and New Trends." *Nutrients* 12, no. 2 (2020): 579. https://doi.org/10.3390/nu12020579.

Rahman, S.M.E., Mahmuda Akter Mele, Young-Tack Lee, and Mohammad Zahirul Islam. "Consumer Preference, Quality, and Safety of Organic and Conventional Fresh Fruits, Vegetables, and Cereals." *Foods* 10, no. 1 (2021): 105. https://doi.org/10.3390/foods10010105.

Rawson, Eric S., Mary P. Miles, and D. Enette Larson-Meyer. "Dietary Supplements for Health, Adaptation, and Recovery in Athletes." *International Journal of Sport Nutrition and Exercise Metabolism* 28, no. 2 (2018): 188–99. https://doi.org/10.1123/ijsnem.2017-0340.

Reynolds, Andrew N., Ashley P. Akerman, and Jim Mann. "Dietary Fibre and Whole Grains in Diabetes Management: Systematic Review and Meta-Analyses." Edited by Ronald Ching Wan Ma. *PLOS Medicine* 17, no. 3 (2020): e1003053. https://doi.org/10.1371/journal.pmed.1003053.

Ross, A, Christine Taylor, Ann Yaktine, and Heather Del Valle. "Dri Dietary Reference Intakes Calcium Vitamin D Committee to Review Dietary Reference Intakes for Vitamin D and Calcium Food and Nutrition Board." (2001).

Sandford, Gareth N., and Trent Stellingwerff. "'Question Your Categories': The Misunderstood Complexity of Middle-Distance Running Profiles with Implications for Research Methods and Application." *Frontiers in Sports and Active Living* 1 (September 2019). https://doi.org/10.3389/fspor.2019.00028.

Saunders, Bryan, Kirsty Elliott-Sale, Guilherme G Artioli, Paul A Swinton, Eimear Dolan, Hamilton Roschel, Craig Sale, and Bruno Gualano. "β-Alanine Supplementation to Improve Exercise Capacity and Performance: A Systematic Review and Meta-Analysis." *British Journal of Sports Medicine* 51, no. 8 (2016): 658–69. https://doi.org/10.1136/bjsports-2016-096396.

Sawka, Michael N., Samuel N. Cheuvront, and Robert W. Kenefick. "Hypohydration and Human Performance: Impact of Environment and Physiological Mechanisms." *Sports Medicine* 45, no. 1 (2015): 51–60. https://doi.org/10.1007/s40279-015-0395-7.

Schoenfeld, Brad Jon, and Alan Albert Aragon. "How Much Protein Can the Body Use in a Single Meal for Muscle-Building? Implications for Daily Protein Distribution." *Journal of the International Society of Sports Nutrition* 15, no. 1 (2018). https://doi.org/10.1186/s12970-018-0215-1.

Shriver, Lenka H., Nancy M. Betts, and Gena Wollenberg. 2013. "Dietary Intakes and Eating Habits of College Athletes: Are Female College Athletes Following the Current Sports Nutrition Standards?" *Journal of American College Health* 61, no. 1 (2013): 10–16. https://doi.org/10.1080/07448481.2012.747526.

Southward, Kyle, Kay J. Rutherfurd-Markwick, and Ajmol Ali. 2018. "The Effect of Acute Caffeine Ingestion on Endurance Performance: A Systematic Review and Meta–Analysis." *Sports Medicine* 48, no. 8 (2018): 1913–28. https://doi.org/10.1007/s40279-018-0939-8.

Suhett, Lara Gomes, Rodrigo de Miranda Monteiro Santos, Brenda Kelly Souza Silveira, Arieta Carla Gualandi Leal, Alice Divina Melo de Brito, Juliana Farias de Novaes, and Ceres Mattos Della Lucia. "Effects of Curcumin Supplementation on Sport and Physical Exercise: A Systematic Review." *Critical Reviews in Food Science and Nutrition*, (April, 2020). https://doi.org/10.1080/10408398.2020.1749025.

Tanabe, Yoko, Kentaro Chino, Hiroyuki Sagayama, Hyun Jin Lee, Hitomi Ozawa, Seiji Maeda, and Hideyuki Takahashi. "Effective Timing of Curcumin Ingestion to Attenuate Eccentric Exercise-Induced Muscle Soreness in Men." *Journal of Nutritional Science and Vitaminology* 65, no. 1 (2019): 82–89. https://doi.org/10.3177/jnsv.65.82.

Tanabe, Yoko, Kentaro Chino, Takahiro Ohnishi, Hitomi Ozawa, Hiroyuki Sagayama, Seiji Maeda, and Hideyuki Takahashi. "Effects of Oral Curcumin Ingested before or after Eccentric Exercise on Markers of Muscle Damage and Inflammation." *Scandinavian Journal of Medicine & Science in Sports* 29, no. 4 (2019): 524–34. https://doi.org/10.1111/sms.13373.

Telford, R. D., G. J. Sly, A. G. Hahn, R. B. Cunningham, C. Bryant, and J. A. Smith. "Footstrike Is the Major Cause of Hemolysis during Running." *Journal of Applied Physiology* 94, no. 1 (2003): 38–42. https://doi.org/10.1152/japplphysiol.00631.2001.

Torres-McGehee, Toni M., Kelly L. Pritchett, Deborah Zippel, Dawn M. Minton, Adam Cellamare, and Mike Sibilia. "Sports Nutrition Knowledge among Collegiate Athletes, Coaches, Athletic Trainers, and Strength and Conditioning Specialists." *Journal of Athletic Training* 47, no. 2 (2012): 205–11. https://doi.org/10.4085/1062-6050-47.2.205.

Van Loon, Luc, Paul Greenhaff, D Constantin-Teodosiu, Wim Saris, and Anton Wagenmakers. "The Effects of Increasing Exercise Intensity on Muscle Fuel Utilisation in Humans." *Journal of Physiology*. (2001).

Vieira, Samantha A, David Julian McClements, and Eric A Decker. "Challenges of Utilizing Healthy Fats in Foods." *Advances in Nutrition* 6, no. 3 (2015): 309S317S. https://doi.org/10.3945/an.114.006965.

Volek, Jeff S, and Eric S Rawson. "Scientific Basis and Practical Aspects of Creatine Supplementation for Athletes." *Nutrition* 20, no. 7-8 (2004): 609–14. https://doi.org/10.1016/j.nut.2004.04.014.

## CHP. 3

Ansari, Walid, Hamed Adetunji, and Reza Oskrochi. "Food and Mental Health: Relationship between Food and Perceived Stress and Depressive Symptoms among University Students in the United Kingdom." *Cent Eur J Public Health* 22, no. 2 (2014): 90–97.

Carbone, John W, James P McClung, and Stefan M Pasiakos. "Recent Advances in the Characterization of Skeletal Muscle and Whole-Body Protein Responses to Dietary Protein and Exercise during Negative Energy Balance." *Advances in Nutrition* 10, no. 1 (2018): 70–79. https://doi.org/10.1093/advances/nmy087.

Cava, Edda, Nai Chien Yeat, and Bettina Mittendorfer. "Preserving Healthy Muscle during Weight Loss." *Advances in Nutrition: An International Review Journal* 8, no. 3 (2017): 511–19. https://doi.org/10.3945/an.116.014506.

Chu, Yen Li, Anna Farmer, Christina Fung, Stefan Kuhle, Kate E Storey, and Paul J Veugelers. "Involvement in Home Meal Preparation Is Associated with Food Preference and Self-Efficacy among Canadian Children." *Public Health Nutrition* 16, no. 1 (2012): 108–12. https://doi.org/10.1017/s1368980012001218.

Cuenca-Sánchez, Marta, Diana Navas-Carrillo, and Esteban Orenes-Piñero. "Controversies Surrounding High-Protein Diet Intake: Satiating Effect and Kidney and Bone Health." *Advances in Nutrition* 6, no. 3 (2015): 260–66. https://doi.org/10.3945/an.114.007716.

Flanagan, Shalane, Elyse Kopecky, and Alan Weiner. *Run Fast. Eat Slow: Nourishing Recipes for Athletes*. Emmaus, Pennsylvania: Rodale, 2016.

Hartmann, Christina, Simone Dohle, and Michael Siegrist. "Importance of Cooking Skills for Balanced Food Choices." *Appetite* 65 (June 2013):125–31. https://doi.org/10.1016/j.appet.2013.01.016.

Larson, Nicole I., Cheryl L. Perry, Mary Story, and Dianne Neumark-Sztainer. "Food Preparation by Young Adults Is Associated with Better Diet Quality." *Journal of the American Dietetic Association* 106, no. 12 (2006): 2001–7. https://doi.org/10.1016/j.jada.2006.09.008.

Layman, Donald K. "Dietary Guidelines Should Reflect New Understandings about Adult Protein Needs." *Nutrition & Metabolism* 6, no. 1 (2009): 12. https://doi.org/10.1186/1743-7075-6-12.

Mclaughlin, Carey, Valerie Tarasuk, and Nancy Kreiger. "An Examination of At-Home Food Preparation Activity among Low-Income, Food-Insecure Women." *Journal of the American Dietetic Association* 103, no. 1 (2003): 1506–12. https://doi.org/10.1016/j.jada.2003.08.022.

Monsivais, Pablo, Anju Aggarwal, and Adam Drewnowski. "Time Spent on Home Food Preparation and Indicators of Healthy Eating." *American Journal of Preventive Medicine* 47, no. 6 (2014): 796–802. https://doi.org/10.1016/j.amepre.2014.07.033.

Smith, Lindsey P, Shu Wen Ng, and Barry M Popkin. "Trends in US Home Food Preparation and Consumption: Analysis of

National Nutrition Surveys and Time Use Studies from 1965–1966 to 2007–2008." *Nutrition Journal* 12, no. 1 (2013). https://doi.org/10.1186/1475-2891-12-45.

Zick, Cathleen D, and Robert B Stevens. "Trends in Americans' Food-Related Time Use: 1975–2006." *Public Health Nutrition* 13, no. 7 (2009): 1064–72. https://doi.org/10.1017/s1368980009992138.

## CHP. 4

Afaghi, Ahmad, Helen O'Connor, and Chin Moi Chow. "High-Glycemic-Index Carbohydrate Meals Shorten Sleep Onset." *The American Journal of Clinical Nutrition* 85, no. 2 (2007): 426–30. https://doi.org/10.1093/ajcn/85.2.426.

Ahmed, Will (@willahmed). "You want to sleep better but you don't have more time to spend in bed. OK, no problem I've spent 10 years researching sleep as an athlete then and entrepreneur and of course as a founder of @whoop […]." Twitter, March 2, 2021. 9:08 a.m. https://twitter.com/willahmed/status/1366752177704865795.

Alahmary, Sarah, Sakinah Alduhaylib, Hibah Alkawii, Mashail Olwani, Reem Shablan, Hala Ayoub, Tunny Purayidathil, Omar Abuzaid, and Rabie Khattab. "Relationship between Added Sugar Intake and Sleep Quality among University Students: A Cross-Sectional Study." *American Journal of Lifestyle Medicine*, February 2019.

Belenky, Gregory, Nancy J. Wesensten, David R. Thorne, Maria L. Thomas, Helen C. Sing, Daniel P. Redmond, Michael B. Russo, and Thomas J. Balkin. "Patterns of Performance Degradation and Restoration during Sleep Restriction and Subsequent Recovery: A Sleep Dose-Response Study." *Journal of Sleep Research* 12, no.1 (2003): 1–12. https://doi.org/10.1046/j.1365-2869.2003.00337.x.

Breus, Michael. Psychology Today. "5 Ways That Vitamin Deficiencies Can Impact Your Sleep." *Sleep Newzzz.* May 30, 2019. https://www.psychologytoday.com/us/blog/sleep-newzzz/201905/5-ways-vitamin-deficiencies-can-impact-your-sleep.

Cain, Neralie, and Michael Gradisar. "Electronic Media Use and Sleep in School-Aged Children and Adolescents: A Review." *Sleep Medicine* 11, no. 8 (2010): 735–42. https://doi.org/10.1016/j.sleep.2010.02.006.

Dewald, Julia F., Anne M. Meijer, Frans J. Oort, Gerard A. Kerkhof, and Susan M. Bögels. "The Influence of Sleep Quality, Sleep Duration and Sleepiness on School Performance in Children and Adolescents: A Meta-Analytic Review." *Sleep Medicine Reviews* 14, no. 3 (2010): 179–89. https://doi.org/10.1016/j.smrv.2009.10.004.

Djokic, Gorica, Petar Vojvodic, Davor Korcok, Anita Agic, Anica Rankovic, Vladan Djordjevic, Aleksandra Vojvodic, et al. "The Effects of Magnesium – Melatonin - Vit B Complex Supplementation in Treatment of Insomnia." *Open Access Macedonian Journal of Medical Sciences* 7, no. 18 (2019): 3101–5. https://doi.org/10.3889/oamjms.2019.771.

Finestone, Aharon, and Charles Milgrom. "How Stress Fracture Incidence Was Lowered in the Israeli Army." *Medicine & Sci-*

*ence in Sports & Exercise* 40, no. 11 (2008): S623–29. https://doi. org/10.1249/mss.0b013e3181892dc2.

Fullagar, Hugh H K, Sabrina Skorski, Rob Duffield, Daniel Hammes, Aaron J Coutts, and Tim Meyer. "Sleep and Athletic Performance: The Effects of Sleep Loss on Exercise Performance, and Physiological and Cognitive Responses to Exercise." *Sports Medicine (Auckland, N.Z.)* 45, no. 2 (2015): 161–86. https:// doi.org/10.1007/s40279-014-0260-0.

Gordon, Ian. Mother Jones. "Minor League Baseball Players Make Poverty-Level Wages". *Politics.* July 2014. https://www. motherjones.com/politics/2014/06/baseball-broshuis-mi-nor-league-wage-income/

Howatson, Glyn, Phillip G. Bell, Jamie Tallent, Benita Middleton, Malachy P. McHugh, and Jason Ellis. "Effect of Tart Cherry Juice (Prunus Cerasus) on Melatonin Levels and Enhanced Sleep Quality." *European Journal of Nutrition* 51, no. 8 (2011): 909–16. https://doi.org/10.1007/s00394-011-0263-7.

Jäger, Ralf, Chad M. Kerksick, Bill I. Campbell, Paul J. Cribb, Shawn D. Wells, Tim M. Skwiat, Martin Purpura, et al. "International Society of Sports Nutrition Position Stand: Protein and Exercise." *Journal of the International Society of Sports Nutrition* 14, no. 1 (2017). https://doi.org/10.1186/s12970-017-0177-8.

Lindseth, Glenda, Paul Lindseth, and Mark Thompson. "Nutritional Effects on Sleep." *Western Journal of Nursing Research* 35, no. 4 (2013): 497–513. https://doi.org/10.1177/0193945911416379.

Mah, Cheri D., Eric J. Kezirian, Brandon M. Marcello, and William C. Dement. "Poor Sleep Quality and Insufficient Sleep of a Collegiate Student-Athlete Population." *Sleep Health* 4, no. 3 (2018): 251–57. https://doi.org/10.1016/j.sleh.2018.02.005.

Mah, Cheri D., Kenneth E. Mah, Eric J. Kezirian, and William C. Dement. "The Effects of Sleep Extension on the Athletic Performance of Collegiate Basketball Players." *Sleep* 34, no. 7 (2011): 943–50. https://doi.org/10.5665/sleep.1132.

Milewski, Matthew D., David L. Skaggs, Gregory A. Bishop, J. Lee Pace, David A. Ibrahim, Tishya A.L. Wren, and Audrius Barzdukas. "Chronic Lack of Sleep Is Associated with Increased Sports Injuries in Adolescent Athletes." *Journal of Pediatric Orthopaedics* 34, no. 2 (2014): 129–33. https://doi.org/10.1097/bpo.0000000000000151.

Moore, Melisa, and Lisa J. Meltzer. "The Sleepy Adolescent: Causes and Consequences of Sleepiness in Teens." *Paediatric Respiratory Reviews* 9, no. 2 (2008): 114–21. https://doi.org/10.1016/j.prrv.2008.01.001.

Pigeon, Wilfred R., Michelle Carr, Colin Gorman, and Michael L. Perlis. "Effects of a Tart Cherry Juice Beverage on the Sleep of Older Adults with Insomnia: A Pilot Study." *Journal of Medicinal Food* 13, no. 3. (2010): 579–83. https://doi.org/10.1089/jmf.2009.0096.

Reilly, Thomas, and Mark Piercy. "The Effect of Partial Sleep Deprivation on Weight-Lifting Performance." *Ergonomics* 37, no. 1 (1994): 107–15. https://doi.org/10.1080/00140139408963628.

Res, Peter T., Bart Groe, Bart Pennings, Milou Beelen, Gareth A. Wallis, Annemarie P. Gijsen, Joan M. G. Senden and Luc J. C. Van Loon. "Protein Ingestion before Sleep Improves Postexercise Overnight Recovery." *Medicine & Science in Sports & Exercise* 44, no. 8 (2012): 1560–69. https://doi.org/10.1249/mss.0b013e31824cc363.

Snijders, Tim, Joshua P. Nederveen, Kirsten E. Bell, Sean W. Lau, Nicole Mazara, Dinesh A. Kumbhare, Stuart M. Phillips, and Gianni Parise. "Prolonged Exercise Training Improves the Acute Type II Muscle Fibre Satellite Cell Response in Healthy Older Men." *The Journal of Physiology* 597, no. 1 (2018): 105–19. https://doi.org/10.1113/jp276260.

Strand, Bradford, and Andrew Fitzgerald. "The Impact of Sleep on Youth Athletic Performance Leadership and Professional Development View Project Coaching Education View Project." (2015).

Vlahoyiannis, Angelos, Christoforos D. Giannaki, Giorgos K. Sakkas, George Aphamis, and Eleni Andreou. "A Systematic Review, Meta-Analysis and Meta-Regression on the Effects of Carbohydrates on Sleep." *Nutrients* 13, no. 4 (2021): 1283. https://doi.org/10.3390/nu13041283.

Volpe, Stella Lucia. "Magnesium and the Athlete." *Current Sports Medicine Reports* 14, no. 4 (2015): 279–83. https://doi.org/10.1249/jsr.0000000000000178.

Watson, Andrew M. "Sleep and Athletic Performance." *Current Sports Medicine Reports* 16, no. 6 (2017): 413–18. https://doi.org/10.1249/jsr.0000000000000418.

## CHP. 5

Donovan, Nancy J., and Dan Blazer. "Social Isolation and Loneliness in Older Adults: Review and Commentary of a National Academies Report." *The American Journal of Geriatric Psychiatry* 28, no. 12 (2020): 1233–44. https://doi.org/10.1016/j.jagp.2020.08.005.

Levine, Martha Peaslee. "Loneliness and Eating Disorders." *The Journal of Psychology* 146, no. 1-2 (2012): 243–57. https://doi.org/10.1080/00223980.2011.606435.

Lim, Allen, and Biju Thomas. 2016. *Feed Zone Table: Family-Style to Nourish Life and Sport.* VeloPress.

Merriam-Webster.com. s.v "doping." Accessed 2019. http://Merrium-Webster.com.

Sundgot-Borgen, Jorunn, and Monica Klungland Torstveit. "Prevalence of Eating Disorders in Elite Athletes Is Higher than in the General Population." *Clinical Journal of Sport Medicine* 14, no. 1 (2004): 25–32. https://doi.org/10.1097/00042752-200401000-00005.

## CHP. 6

Adeva-Andany, María M., Manuel González-Lucán, Cristóbal Donapetry-García, Carlos Fernández-Fernández, and Eva Ameneiros-Rodríguez."Glycogen Metabolism in Humans." *BBA Clinical* 5 (June 2016): 85–100. https://doi.org/10.1016/j.bbacli.2016.02.001.

Agel, Julie, Atc Ma, Jack Ransone, Randall Dick, Robert Oppliger, and Stephen Marshall. "Descriptive Epidemiology of Collegiate Men's Wrestling Injuries: National Collegiate Athletic Association Injury Surveillance System, 1988-1989 through 2003-2004." *Journal of Athletic Training 303 Journal of Athletic Training* 42, no. 2 (2007): 303–10.

Macdiarmid, JI, and JE Blundell. "Dietary Under-Reporting: What People Say about Recording Their Food Intake." *European Journal of Clinical Nutrition* 51, no. 3 (1997): 199–200. https://doi.org/10.1038/sj.ejcn.1600380.

Mettler, Samuel, Nigel Mitchell, and Kevin D. Tipton. "Increased Protein Intake Reduces Lean Body Mass Loss during Weight Loss in Athletes." *Medicine & Science in Sports & Exercise* 42, no. 2 (2010): 326–37. https://doi.org/10.1249/mss.0b013e-3181b2ef8e.

Tipton, Kevin D. "Nutritional Support for Exercise-Induced Injuries." *Sports Medicine* 45, no.1 (2015): 93–104. https://doi.org/10.1007/s40279-015-0398-4.

Waters, Robert L., Joyce Campbell, and Jacquelin Perry. "Energy Cost of Three-Point Crutch Ambulation in Fracture Patients." *Journal of Orthopaedic Trauma* 1, no. 2 (1987): 170–73. https://doi.org/10.1097/00005131-198702010-00007.

World Health Organization. "World Health Organization." Who.int. World Health Organization. 2022. https://www.who.int/.

Worsley, A., W. Coonan, P.A. Baghurst, M. Peters, and A.J. Worsley. 1984. "Australian Ten Year Olds' Perceptions of Foods: II.

Social Status Effects." *Ecology of Food and Nutrition* 15, no. 3 (1984): 247–57. https://doi.org/10.1080/03670244.1984.9990831.


**CHP. 7**

Ain, Morty. ESPN.com. "Colts O-Linemen Embody Evolution of the Position." July 6, 2015. https://www.espn.com/nfl/story/_/page/bodycoltsoline/indianapolis-colts-offensive-linemen-embody-evolution-position-espn-magazine-body-issue.

Burtka, Jeff. GlobalSport Matters. "Body Image Issues Can Impact Athletes at a Young Age." *Health.* September 20, 2019. https://globalsportmatters.com/health/2019/09/20/body-image-issues-can-impact-athletes-at-a-young-age/.

Burtka, Jeff. GlobalSport Matters. "Hidden figures: Male athlete eating disorders often overlooked." *Health.* August 28, 2019. https://globalsportmatters.com/health/2019/09/20/body-image-issues-can-impact-athletes-at-a-young-age/.

Chatterton, Justine M., and Trent A. Petrie. "Prevalence of Disordered Eating and Pathogenic Weight Control Behaviors among Male Collegiate Athletes." *Eating Disorders* 21, no. 4 (2013): 328–41. https://doi.org/10.1080/10640266.2013.797822.

Clifford, Tom, and Charlotte Blyth. "A Pilot Study Comparing the Prevalence of Orthorexia Nervosa in Regular Students and Those in University Sports Teams." *Eating and Weight Disorders - Studies on Anorexia, Bulimia and Obesity* 24, no. 3 (2018): 473–80. https://doi.org/10.1007/s40519-018-0584-0.

Grace, Kate. "Race Weight." Training Notes (blog). February 13, 2019. https://fastk8.com/2019/02/13/race-weight/.

Futterman, Matthew. The New York Times. "Jessie Diggins Wins Bronze in the Individual Sprint, Her Second Olympic Medal." *Sports.* February 8, 2022, https://www.nytimes.com/2022/02/07/sports/olympics/jessie-diggins-bronze-sprint-cross-country.html?.

Joy, Elizabeth, Andrea Kussman, and Aurelia Nattiv. "2016 Update on Eating Disorders in Athletes: A Comprehensive Narrative Review with a Focus on Clinical Assessment and Management." *British Journal of Sports Medicine* 50, no. 3 (2016): 154–62. https://doi.org/10.1136/bjsports-2015-095735.

Ouyang, Yiyi, Kun Wang, Tingran Zhang, Li Peng, Gan Song, and Jiong Luo. "The Influence of Sports Participation on Body Image, Self-Efficacy, and Self-Esteem in College Students." *Frontiers in Psychology* 10 (February 2020). https://doi.org/10.3389/fpsyg.2019.03039.

Parker, Kayla. "How April Ross Got That Body." ESPN.com .July 6, 2016. https://www.espn.com/espnw/life-style/story/_/id/16822841/how-beach-volleyball-olympian-april-ross-got-body.

Petrie, Trent A., Christy Greenleaf, Justine Reel, and Jennifer Carter. 2009. "Personality and Psychological Factors as Predictors of Disordered Eating among Female Collegiate Athletes." *Eating Disorders* 17, no. 4 (2009): 302–21. https://doi.org/10.1080/10640260902991160.

Power, Ksenia, Sara Kovacs, Lois Butcher-Poffley, Jingwei Wu, and David Sarwer. 2020. "Disordered Eating and Compulsive Exercise in Collegiate Athletes: Applications for Sport and Research. Thesportjournal.org/Article/Disordered-Eating-And-Compulsive-Exercise-In-Collegiate-Athletes-Applications-For-Sport-And- Research Disordered Eating and Compulsive Exercise in Collegiate Athletes: Applications for Sport and Research."

Soulliard, Zachary A., Alicia A. Kauffman, Hannah F. Fitterman-Harris, Joanne E. Perry, and Michael J. Ross. "Examining Positive Body Image, Sport Confidence, Flow State, and Subjective Performance among Student Athletes and Non-Athletes." *Body Image* 28 (March 2019): 93–100. https://doi.org/10.1016/j.bodyim.2018.12.009.

Steinfeldt, Jesse A., Rebecca A. Zakrajsek, Kimberly J. Bodey, Katharine G. Middendorf, and Scott B. Martin. "Role of Uniforms in the Body Image of Female College Volleyball Players." *The Counseling Psychologist* 41, no. 5 (2012): 791–819. https://doi.org/10.1177/0011000012457218.

Team USA. "Why Do Some Athletes Struggle with Body Image?". News. 2022. https://www.teamusa.org/USA-Softball/News/2020/June/01/Why-Do-Some-Athletes-Struggle-with-Body-Image.

Tod, David, Leuan Cranswick, and Christian Edwards. "Muscle Dysmorphia: Current Insights beyond the Muscles: Exploring the Role of the Drive for Muscularity in Identity. View Project." *Psychology Research and Behavior Management* 9 (2016). https://doi.org/10.2147/PRBM.S97404.

Torstveit, M. K., J. H. Rosenvinge, and J. Sundgot-Borgen. "Prevalence of Eating Disorders and the Predictive Power of Risk Models in Female Elite Athletes: A Controlled Study." *Scandinavian Journal of Medicine & Science in Sports* 18, no. 1 (2007): 108–18. https://doi.org/10.1111/j.1600-0838.2007.00657.x.

**CHP. 8**

Cranny, Elise and Stef Strack. "Elise Cranny Fuel Your Body & Mind September, 21 2020. in *Voice In Sport*. Produced by Liz Boyer and Anya Miller. Podcast, MP3 audio, 26.16 https://www.voiceinsport.com/tune_in/podcast/fuel-your-body-and-mind.

Dictionary.com. s.v. "health food." Accessed June 3, 2022. https://www.dictionary.com/.

Johnson, Craig, Pauline Powers, and Randy Dick. "Athletes and Eating Disorders: The National Collegiate Athletic Association Study." *International Journal of Eating Disorders* 26, no. 2 (1999).

Lyons, Libby. 2018. "UC San Diego 4th Annual Eating Disorders Conference Innovative Treatments." Eating Disorder Hope. January 24, 2018. https://www.eatingdisorderhope.com/blog/orthorexia-athletes-die-disorder.

Medrano, Megan. 2019. "WHEN HEALTHY EATING GOES TOO FAR: THE LINK between ORTHOREXIA and ATHLETES." WellSeek. September 30, 2019. https://wellseek.co/2019/09/30/when-healthy-eating-goes-too-far-the-link-between-orthorexia-and-athlete/.

National Eating Disorders Association. "Orthorexia." *Information by Eating Disorder.* February 22, 2018. https://www.nationaleatingdisorders.org/learn/by-eating-disorder/other/orthorexia.

Run Whole Nutrition. *Home.* 2021. https://www.runwholenutrition.com/.

Segura-Garcia, Christina, Maria Papaianni, Francesca Caglioti, Leonardo Procopio, Cristiano Nistico, Luca Bombardiere, Antonio Ammendolia, et al. "Orthorexia Nervosa: A Frequent Eating Disordered Behavior in Athletes." *Eating and Weight Disorders* 17, no. 4 (2012).